THE CARE OF WOUNDS
A GUIDE FOR NURSES

CAROL DEALEY BSc (Hons), RGN, RCNT

Clinical Nurse Specialist in Tissue Viability
Queen Elizabeth Hospital, The Community Hospital Division
South Birmingham Health Authority

OXFORD

BLACKWELL SCIENTIFIC PUBLICATIONS

LONDON EDINBURGH BOSTON

MELBOURNE PARIS BERLIN VIENNA

© 1994 by
Blackwell Scientific Publications
Editorial Offices:
Osney Mead, Oxford OX2 0EL
25 John Street, London WC1N 2BL
23 Ainslie Place, Edinburgh EH3 6AJ
238 Main Street, Cambridge,
   Massachusetts 02142, USA
54 University Street, Carlton,
   Victoria 3053, Australia

Other Editorial Offices:
Librairie Arnette SA
1, rue de Lille
75007 Paris
France

Blackwell Wissenschafts-Verlag GmbH
Düsseldorfer Str. 38
D-10707 Berlin
Germany

Blackwell MZV
Feldgasse 13
A-1238 Wien
Austria

First published 1994

Set by DP Photosetting, Aylesbury, Bucks
Printed and bound in Great Britain by
Hartnolls Ltd., Bodmin, Cornwall

DISTRIBUTORS
Marston Book Services Ltd
PO Box 87
Oxford OX2 0DT
(Orders: Tel: 0865 791155
        Fax: 0865 791927
        Telex: 837515)

USA
Blackwell Scientific Publications Inc.
238 Main Street
Cambridge, MA 02142
(Orders: Tel: 800 759-6102
              617 876-7000)

Canada
Times Mirror Professional Publishing Ltd
130 Flaska Drive
Markham, Ontario L6G 1B8
(Orders: Tel: 800 268-4178
              416 470-6739)

Australia
Blackwell Scientific Publications Pty Ltd
54 University Street,
Carlton, Victoria 3053
(Orders: Tel: 03 347-5552)

British Library
Cataloguing in Publication Data
A Catalogue record for this book is available from the
British Library

ISBN 0–632–03864–0

Library of Congress
Cataloging in Publication Data
Dealey, Carol.
      The care of wounds: a guide for nurses/
Carol Dealey.
         p.   cm.
      Includes bibliographical references and index.
      ISBN 0–632–03864–0
      1. Wounds and injuries–Nursing.   2. Wound
healing.   I. Title.
      [DNLM: 1. Wounds and Injuries–nursing.
2. Wound Healing–physiology.
WO 700 D279c   1994]
RD93.95.D43   1994
617.1–dc20
DNLM/DLC
for Library of Congress   93-47189
                                                  CIP

Contents

Preface

Wound management is a fascinating and rewarding subject. I became involved in it some years ago and still get a sense of excitement at the challenge of dealing with any case of problematic wound healing. Much progress has been made in the last few years and there is still more to discover. As medicine becomes more and more sophisticated, so wound care can seem correspondingly complex. The wide range of choices available for wound management can cause considerable confusion for many nurses. The purpose of this book is to clarify some of the areas of confusion and to provide clear guidelines for consistent wound management. It is intended for any nurse who cares for patients with wounds.

I would like to thank the many people who have helped me in preparing this book, not least my patients, from whom I have learnt a great deal. However, I must thank my family most of all, for giving up the time that I should have spent with them in order for me to write this.

Carol Dealey

Chapter 1
The Physiology of Wound Healing

Wound healing is a highly complex process. It is important that the nurse has an understanding of the physiological processes involved. This is for several reasons:

(1) An understanding of normal physiology enables the nurse to recognize the abnormal.
(2) Recognition of the stages of healing allows the nurse to select appropriate dressings.
(3) Understanding of the requirements of the healing process means that appropriate nutrition can, as far as is possible, be given to the patient.

1.1 INTRODUCTION

The wound healing process consists of a series of highly complex, interdependent, and overlapping stages. These stages have been given a variety of names. They are described here as:

- Inflammation
- Reconstruction
- Epithelialization
- Maturation

The stages last for variable lengths of time. Any stage may be prolonged because of local factors such as ischaemia or lack of nutrients. The factors which can delay healing are discussed in more detail in Chapter 3.

Any damage leading to a break in the continuity of the skin can be called a wound. There are several causes of wounding:

- *Trauma* – mechanical, chemical, physical
- *Surgery*
- *Ischaemia* – e.g. arterial leg ulcer
- *Pressure* – e.g. pressure sore

In both traumatic and surgical (i.e. intentional) injury there is rupture of blood vessels which results in bleeding, followed by clot formation. In wounds caused by ischaemia or pressure the blood supply is disrupted by local occlusion of the microcirculation. Tissue necrosis follows and results in ulcer formation, possibly with a necrotic eschar or scab.

Wounds in the skin or deeper tissues have been labelled in various ways. Some of them can be described as follows:

(1) *Partial- and full-thickness wounds* In a partial-thickness wound, some of the dermis remains and there are shafts of hair follicles or sweat glands. In a full-thickness wound all the dermis is destroyed and deeper layers may also be involved.

(2) *Healing by first and second intention* First described by Hippocrates around 350 BC.
   (a) healing by first intention is when there is no tissue loss and the skin edges are held in apposition to each other, such as a sutured wound;
   (b) healing by second intention means a wound where there has been tissue loss and the skin edges are far apart, such as a leg ulcer;

(3) *Open and closed wounds* These are the same as healing by second and first intention, respectively.

1.2 INFLAMMATION

The inflammatory response is a non-specific local reaction to tissue damage and/or bacterial invasion. It is an important part of the body's defence mechanisms and is an essential part of the healing process. The signs of inflammation were first described by Celsus in AD 100 as redness, heat, pain and swelling. The factors causing them are shown in Table 1.1.

Tissue damage triggers both the complement and kinin systems. The complement system consists of plasma proteins which are inactive precursors. When activated, there is a cascade effect which leads to the release of histamine from the mast cells and results in vasodilation and increased capillary permeability. This effect is enhanced by the kinin system which, through a series of steps, activates kininogen to kinins. Kinins have several other effects. They attract neutrophils to the wound, enhance phagocytosis and cause pain by stimulating the sensory nerve endings.

As the capillaries dilate and become more permeable, fluid flows into the injured tissues. This fluid then becomes the 'inflammatory exudate', and it contains plasma proteins, antibodies, red and white blood cells (erythrocytes and leucocytes) and

Table 1.1 The signs of inflammation.

Signs and symptoms	Physiological rationale
Redness	Large amount of blood in the area following vasodilation.
Heat	Large amount of warm blood and heat energy produced by metabolic reactions.
Swelling	Presence of fluid in the tissues surrounding the wound.
Pain	May be caused by damage to nerve endings, activation of the kinin system, pressure of fluid in the tissues or the presence of enzymes, such as prostaglandins, which cause chemical irritation.

platelets. As well as being involved in clot formation, platelets also release growth factors and fibronectin. Their role is to promote cell migration and growth at the wound site.

The first leucocyte to arrive at the wound is the neutrophil. Wagner (1985) has described the role of fibronectin in relation to neutrophils. It attracts neutrophils to the wound site – a process known as chemotaxis. Neutrophils squeeze through the capillary walls into the tissues by diapedesis, again this ability is enhanced by fibronectin. Within about an hour of the inflammatory response being initiated, neutrophils can be found at the wound site. They arrive in large numbers, their role being to phagocytose bacteria by engulfing and destroying them.

Growth factors from the platelets attract monocytes to the wound. Once in the tissues these cells become known as macrophages. They have the same properties of chemotaxis, diapedesis and phagocytosis found in neutrophils. Macrophages are larger than neutrophils and so are able to phagocytose larger particles, such as necrotic debris, as well as bacteria. The lifespan of the neutrophil can be a few hours or a few days. When neutrophils die they are also phagocytosed by the macrophages.

Inflammation lasts about four to five days, and it requires both energy and nutritional resources. In large wounds the requirements may be considerable. If this stage is prolonged by irritation to the wound – such as infection, foreign body or damage caused by the dressing – it can be debilitating to the patient as well as delaying healing.

1.3 RECONSTRUCTION

Macrophages play a pivotal role in moving from inflammation to reconstruction, as shown in Fig. 1.1. They produce growth factors which attract fibroblasts to the wound and stimulate them to divide and later to produce collagen fibres. Fibronectin also seems to play a role in enhancing fibroblast activity (Orgill & Demling, 1988). Collagen has been seen in a new wound as early as the second day. The activity of fibroblasts depends on the local oxygen supply. If the tissues are poorly vascularized the wound will not heal well. Macrophages assist in improving fibroblast activity by stimulating the growth of new blood vessels capable of bringing oxygen to the wound.

The wound surface has a relatively low oxygen tension, encouraging the macrophages to produce angiogenesis factor which instigates the process of angiogenesis – the growth of new blood vessels. Undamaged capillaries beneath the wound sprout buds which grow towards the surface and loop over and back to the capillary. The loops form a network within the wound supplying oxygen and nutrients.

In wounds healing by first intention, little can be seen of this stage of healing. But in those healing by second intention, the wound can be seen to be filled with granulation tissue. It consists of a dense array of macrophages, fibroblasts, capillary buds and loops in a matrix of fibronectin, collagen and hyaluronic acid. Fig. 1.2 demonstrates the microscopic view of the macrophages forming the advance

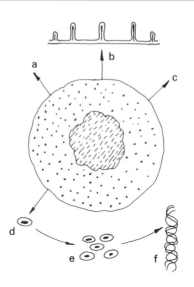

Fig. 1.1 The role of the macrophage: (a) phagocytosis of bacteria, debris and spent neutrophils; (b) stimulates angiogenesis; (c) production of growth factors, e.g. angiogenesis factor; (d) attracts fibroblasts to wound; (e) stimulates cell division; (f) stimulates fibroblasts to produce collagen.

guard, clearing the wound cavity. They are followed by capillary buds growing towards the areas of low oxygen tension in the wound.

Some fibroblasts have a further role: there are specialized fibroblasts, known as myofibroblasts (Gabbiani *et al.*, 1973), which have a contractile apparatus which causes contraction of the wound. It may start at around the fifth or sixth day. Contraction considerably reduces the surface area of open wounds. Irvin (1987)

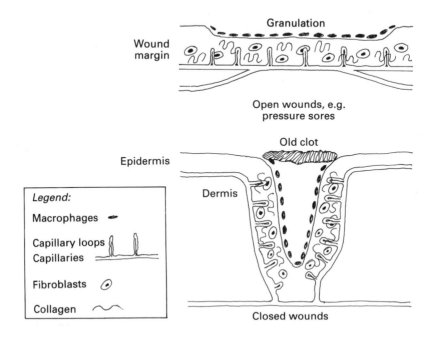

Fig. 1.2 The process of reconstruction in open and closed wounds.

suggests that contraction could be responsible for as much as 40–80% of the closure. It is certainly of considerable importance in large cavity wounds. However, in wounds with a large surface area, such as burns, contraction may lead to contractures.

As the wound fills with new tissue and a capillary network is formed, the number of macrophages and fibroblasts gradually reduces. This stage may have started before the inflammation stage is completed, and prolonged inflammation can result in excessive granulation with hypertrophic scarring. The length of time needed for reconstruction depends on the type and size of wound, but may be about 24 days for wounds healing by first intention.

1.4 EPITHELIALIZATION

This describes the phase where the wound is covered with epithelial cells. The squamous cells at the wound margins and around hair follicle remnants proliferate and migrate over the wound surface in a leap-frog fashion. When cells meet, either in the centre of the wound, forming islets of cells, or at the margin, they stop. This is known as contact inhibition. Epithelial cells only move over viable tissue and require a moist environment (Winter, 1962). In sutured wounds, epithelial cells also migrate along the suture tracks. They are either pulled out with the sutures, or gradually disappear.

This phase commences as early as the second day in closed wounds. However, in open wounds it is necessary for the wound cavity to be filled with granulation tissue before epithelialization can commence. There is a very variable time span for this stage.

1.5 MATURATION

During maturation the wound becomes less vascularized as there is a reduction in the need to bring cells to the wound site. The collagen fibres are re-organized so that, instead of being laid down in a random fashion, they lie at right angles to the wound margins. The scar tissue present is gradually remodelled and becomes comparable to normal tissue after a long period of time. The scar gradually flattens to a thin white line. This takes up to a year in closed wounds and very much longer in open wounds.

Tensile strength gradually increases. This is a way of describing the ability of the wound to resist rupture or dehiscence. Forester et al. (1969) found that at 10 days an apparently well-healed surgical incision has little strength. During maturation it increases so that by three months the tensile strength is 50% that of normal tissue. Further work by Forester et al. (1970) compared surgical incisions where the skin edges were held together by tape with those where sutures were used. The findings showed that, when tape was used, the wounds regained 90% strength of normal tissue, whereas sutured wounds only regained 70% strength.

1.6 CONCLUSION

This section has described 'normal' physiology. However, not all wounds heal without complication or delay. Many factors can affect the healing process. These factors will be considered in more detail in Chapters 3 and 4.

It is also important to recognize that although great strides have been made in the last 10–20 years in the understanding of the healing process, it is still incompletely understood. No doubt, there will be further progress in the next few years.

REFERENCES

Forester, J.C., Zederfeldt, B.H. & Hunt, T.K. (1969) A bioengineering approach to the healing wound. *Journal of Surgical Research* **9**, 207.

Forester, J.C., Zederfeldt, B.H. & Hunt, T.K. (1970) Tape-closed and sutured wounds: a comparison by tensiometry and scanning electron microscope. *British Journal of Surgery* **57**, 729.

Gabbiani, G., Hajno, G.C. & Ryan, G.B. (1973) The fibroblast as a contractile cell: the myofibroblast. In Kulonen, E., Pikkarainen, J. (eds) *The Biology of the Fibroblast*. Academic Press, London.

Irvin, T.T. (1987) The principles of wound healing. *Surgery* **1**, 1112–5.

Orgill, D.G. & Demling, R.H. (1988) Current concepts and approaches to wound healing. *Critical Care Medicine* **16**: 9, 899–908.

Wagner, B.M. (1985) Wound healing revisited: fibronectin and company. *Human Pathology* **16**: 11, 1081.

Winter, G.D. (1962) Formation of the scab and the rate of epithelialization of superficial wounds in the skin of the domestic pig. *Nature* **193**, 293.

Chapter 2
Wound Management Products

2.1 INTRODUCTION

There are many wound management products available and much conflicting advice on how they should be used. Many nurses have a great interest in this subject, and take a justifiable pride in the acquired skills which facilitate dressing change. Recent developments have demonstrated a need to change or adapt traditional practices.

Wound management products include topical agents as well as dressings. A topical agent is that which is applied to a wound. A dressing is a covering on a wound which is intended to promote healing and provide protection from further injury. The Department of Health (DoH) divides dressings into primary and secondary. A primary dressing is that which is used in direct contact with damaged tissue. A secondary dressing is superimposed over the primary dressing.

2.2 THE DEVELOPMENT OF DRESSINGS THROUGH THE AGES

In *L'Ingenue* (1767) Voltaire described history as a 'tableau of crimes and misfortunes'. A study of the dressings used through the ages suggests that there may be some truth in this. Some of the treatments used on the wounded were bizarre, if not horrific, whilst others are still familiar today.

2.2.1 Early history

The earliest record of any dressing can be found on the Edwin Smith Papyrus from Luxor (Zimmerman & Veith, 1961). The papyrus is dated at around 1700 BC, but it is a copy of original manuscripts which date back to around 3000–2500 BC. A variety of dressings are mentioned, including grease, honey, lint, and fresh meat which was valued for its haemostatic properties. Adhesive strapping was made by applying gum to strips of linen (Forrest, 1982).

In ancient Greece Hippocrates (c. 460–377 BC) laid the basis for scientific medicine with his emphasis on careful observation. For the most part, he considered that wounds should be kept clean and dry. He recommended tepid water, wine and vinegar for cleansing wounds. If a wound showed signs of inflammation, he suggested applying a cataplasm or poultice to the area around the wound to soften the tissues and to allow free drainage of pus (Zimmerman & Veith, 1961).

Hippocrates also gave the first definition of healing by first intention, where the skin edges are held in approximation to each other, and secondary intention where there is tissue loss and the skin edges are far apart.

Some of these concepts can also be found in the writings of Sushruta, an Indian surgeon, who describes 14 different types of dressings made from silk, linen, wool and cotton (Zimmerman & Veith, 1961). He also placed great emphasis on the importance of cleanliness.

He differed from Hippocrates on the matter of the most appropriate diet for patients. Sushruta considered meat, normally forbidden to Hindus, an important component, whereas Hippocrates recommended the restriction of food and gave only water to drink to his patients (Zimmerman & Veith, 1961).

At the time of the Roman Empire, oil and wine were commonly applied to wounds. Reference to this is made by the Gospel-writer St Luke in the parable of the Good Samaritan.

Celsus compiled a history of the development of medicine from the time of Hippocrates to AD 100 with great detail of the practices of his time. Although it is believed that Celsus was not a physician, he was the first to give a definition of inflammation. He listed the cardinal signs as redness, heat, pain and swelling; he advocated the cleansing of wounds to remove foreign bodies before suturing; he also expected wounds to suppurate, that is, to form pus (Meade, 1968).

It is, however, Galen who stands out as the person whose work has had lasting impact on wound management. Galen (129–199 AD) worked as the surgeon to the gladiators in Pergamun and later as physician to the Emperor Marcus Aurelius. He wrote many books, some of which survived him and were seen as the ultimate in medical knowledge for many centuries. He is particularly known for his theory of laudable pus (*pus bonem et laudabile*), i.e. that the development of pus is necessary for healing and should, therefore, be actively promoted. Galen found the application of writing ink, cobwebs and Lemnian clay to wounds to be efficacious (Forrest, 1982).

After the fall of the Roman Empire, cultural influence moved eastwards, and the Arab doctors of Islam further developed medicine. However, their wound care was based on Galenic teaching. Various cleansing agents were used at this time. They included turpentine, lizard's dung and pigeon's blood. It is difficult to see the benefit of these substances today. Cooked honey and myrrh were used as astringents to reduce the amount of exudate produced by the wound.

In the Middle Ages the Church taught of the relationship between physical and spiritual health. This resulted in the church having control over many aspects of medicine, such as giving support to Galenic teaching. Thus, the belief in the theory of laudable pus persisted and little advancement was made until the nineteenth century. But, there were a few glimmers in the darkness.

With the discovery of gunpowder, warfare changed. Gunshot wounds were believed to be poisonous. In order to treat them, surgeons began to undertake more amputation of limbs. The standard practice was to use boiling oil to cauterise the stump. Ambrose Paré (1510–90) was a well-practised surgeon in this field. One day he did not have enough boiling oil and applied a mixture of egg yolks, oil of roses and turpentine instead. To his amazement his patients made better progress than usual. He then began to question the benefits of the traditional teaching of laudable pus.

But Paré was still a man of his times: he spent two years trying to bribe another surgeon to reveal the recipe for a special balm made by boiling young puppies in oil of lilies, then adding earthworms.

Another surgeon worthy of mention is Heister (1683–1758). In his *General System of Surgery* he reviewed the range of dressings available, listing sticking plaster, compresses and bandages.

2.2.2 Nineteenth and early twentieth century developments

The Crimean War led to a huge demand for dressings. Various types of dressings were produced in the workhouses which were a source of cheap labour: charpie was made from unravelled cloth; oakum was old rope which had been unpicked and teased into fluff; tow was made from broken, ravelled flax fibres; lint is linen which has been scraped on one side. (The production of this dressing was mechanized.) All of these dressings were washed and re-used many times. They gradually became quite soft, but they were not very absorbent.

The credit for the first absorbent dressing must go to Gamgee (1828–86). He found that cotton wool could be made absorbent by removing the oily matter within it. He then covered the cotton wool with bleached gauze to make dressing pads (Lawrence, 1987). Gamgee tissue is still available today.

During the course of the First World War, more and more severely wounded soldiers had to wait several days before receiving more than a simple field dressing. Many wounds became infected and gangrenous, as a result. Antiseptics were developed to help resolve this problem. In particular, two similar antiseptic solutions came into use. They were Eusol (Edinburgh University Solution of Lime) and Dakin's solution.

At this time, Lumière devised a dressing called *tulle gras*, a gauze impregnated with paraffin. Sphagnum moss was also used as it was found to be twice as absorbent as cotton wool. It could also be impregnated with antiseptics and sterilized. Eupad was a dressing designed for use on leg ulcers. It was a Eusol preparation made up with a mixture of boracic and bleach. Another popular type of dressing was Emplastrums. These were made of white leather spread with a plaster mass, to which some type of medication was often added (Turner, 1986).

2.2.3 The British Pharmaceutical Codices

The first *British Pharmaceutical Codex* was published in 1907. It provided information on all the drugs and medicinal preparations in common use throughout the British Empire. Turner (1986) has reviewed the dressings listed in the earliest British pharmaceutical codices and compared them with more recent lists of dressings in the *British Pharmacopoeia*. He found that the list from 1923 contains much that is familiar today. Table 2.1 compares the 1923 list with the 1980 list, showing that little has changed in the intervening years. Gauzes, cotton wool pads and bandages can be seen as very popular methods of wound care. Turner suggests

Table 2.1 Comparison of surgical dressings 1923 and 1980.

1923		1980	
Gauzes, medicated and unmedicated	(13)	Gauze products	(11)
Cotton wools, medicated and unmedicated	(15)	Cotton wool pads (eye)	(1)
Tows, medicated and unmedicated	(14)	Dressing pads	(2)
Lints, medicated and unmedicated	(8)	Impregnated gauze	(3)
Gauze and cotton tissues	(2)	Gauze and cotton tissues	(2)
Jaconet, oiled silk, etc.	(4)	Ribbon gauze	(3)
Bandages	(9)	Bandages	(15)
Emplastrums	(32)	Adhesive pads	(2)
		Foams	(3)
		Contact layers	(2)
		Absorbent cotton	(2)
		Medicated bandages	(4)

that it is only in the last twenty years that any attempt has been made to design materials that are actually functional. Prior to that, dressings were made from materials that happened to come to hand.

2.3 TRADITIONAL TECHNIQUES

These days, nurses can expect to perform the vast majority of dressings, other than simple first aid treatments applied in the home or work place. But this has not always been the case: originally, dressings were applied by doctors; then medical students, particularly those on surgical wards were trained to change dressings; by the 1930s, the task was given to experienced sisters, and ultimately, it has became a recognized nursing task.

During the 1930s and 1940s, as the care of wounds gradually came into the nursing domain, much mystique became attached to the subject of dressings. This was exaggerated with the development of an aseptic, usually non-touch, dressing technique. Merchant (1988) has reviewed the literature on this subject and has concluded that the procedure that was developed in the 1940s is still being used at the present time, even though most hospitals changed to a central sterile supply system by the early 1970s.

In the early days, large water sterilizers were used for preparing the equipment for an aseptic procedure; one was usually found on every ward. It was the task of the night nurses to boil all the metal bowls, receivers and gallipots ready for the morning dressing round. The dressings were packed in drums and sent to a central point for sterilizing. It was left to the ward sister to choose what went into the drum, commonly gauze squares, cotton wool balls and wadding were used. In many hospitals nurses wore masks and gowns – a practice that has gradually disappeared. Usually two nurses carried out the dressing: a clean nurse and a dirty nurse. Much attention was paid to the position of the equipment on top of the trolley and to the frequency and timing of hand washing.

All wounds were re-dressed once or twice daily. The wound was thoroughly cleaned using cotton wool balls and forceps. The method of wiping across the wound surface varied from hospital to hospital. Fig. 2.1 shows some of the common methods. The Hippocratic principle of keeping wounds clean and dry became adapted to 'allowing wounds to dry up'. Mostly gauze preparations were used, but gradually all sorts of dubious practices crept in. There have been reports of Marmite, eggs, and even toast used on wounds (Johnson, 1987; Dubranski, 1988).

A wide variety of pharmaceutical preparations have also been applied without any recognition of the need for research-based care. Several studies have shown the wide range of dressings being used in different areas. Murray (1988) found that within her health authority an amazing selection of pharmaceutical products were in use: 18 different cleansing agents, 53 substances left in contact with open wounds, and 24 products used for packing wounds. Millward (1989) found 19 different substances being used on pressure sores within one hospital. Walsh & Ford (1989) have discussed the rituals in nursing, many of which can be applied to wound care. The common reasons for choosing a particular dressing could be listed as:

(1) 'We always do it that way here'.
(2) 'Sister said so'.
(3) 'I have used this dressing for the last 30 years, why should I change?'

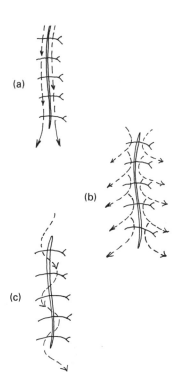

Fig. 2.1 Some of the common methods used for wound cleansing: (a) 'one wipe and away', swabbing along the length of the wound; (b) swabbing in short sweeps away from sutures; (c) rubbing along the length of the wound.

Many nurses will be familiar with these practices, even if they are newcomers to the profession. It is only recently that there has been a critical evaluation of these methods and changes made to more research-based practices. There is a move towards a commonsense approach of seeking to both question procedures and understand what they achieve.

2.4 THE USE OF LOTIONS

A variety of lotions are used in wound care. They are used primarily in wound cleansing. The aims of wound cleansing are to remove any foreign matter, such as gravel or soil, to remove any loose surface debris, such as necrotic tissue, and to remove any remnants of the previous dressing. A study by Thomlinson (1987) considered the various ways that swabs could be wiped across the wound surface. The results showed that the action of cleansing did not reduce the number of bacteria on the wound surface, but simply redistributed them.

2.4.1 Antiseptics

The commonest type of lotion in use is an antiseptic. An antiseptic can be defined as a non-toxic disinfectant which can be applied to skin or living tissues and has the ability to destroy vegetative compounds, such as bacteria, by preventing their growth. If they are used to simply wipe across the wound surface they will have little effect. Antiseptics need to be in contact with bacteria for about twenty minutes before they actually destroy them (Russell *et al.*, 1982). In some instances they can be applied in the form of soaks or incorporated into dressings, ointments or creams.

However, research using experimental wounds in the animal model have demonstrated antiseptics have toxic effects which need to be weighed against any advantages obtained from their use. They have a variety of uses and actions and so are best considered individually.

Cetrimide

This is useful for its detergent properties – particularly in the initial cleansing of traumatic wounds or in the removal of scabs and crusts in skin disease. It should not be used in contact with the eye. It is rapidly inactivated by organic material. Two dangers should be noted, it can cause skin irritation and sensitivity and it is readily contaminated by bacteria, especially *Pseudomonas aeruginosa*. It is mostly only used in accident and emergency departments for initial cleansing of wounds rather than as a routine cleanser.

It is available as a cream or as a lotion in combination with chlorhexidine.

Chlorhexidine

Chlorhexidine is widely used in a variety of aqueous formulations. It is effective against Gram-positive and Gram-negative organisms. Brennan *et al.* (1986) found that it has a low toxicity to living cells. Kearney *et al.* (1988) found that it could maintain its antimicrobial levels for a period of time when impregnated into a dressing. However, the efficacy of chlorhexidine is rapidly diminished in the presence of organic material such as pus or blood (Reynolds, 1982).

Chlorhexidine is sometimes combined with cetrimide.

Hydrogen peroxide 3% (10 vols)

This has an oxidizing effect which destroys anaerobic bacteria. However, it loses its effect when it comes in contact with organic material such as pus or cotton gauze. The oxidizing effect is also beneficial in removing slough from wounds. A study by Graber *et al.* (1975) found that hydrogen peroxide assisted in the rapid removal of slough, but, if it was used on a granulating wound, air blisters formed which burst and led to further breakdown of the wound.

Lineaweaver *et al.* (1985) showed that hydrogen peroxide was cytotoxic to fibroblasts unless diluted to a strength of 0.003%. This dilution is not effective against bacteria. There is also a report of an incident where an air embolism occurred after irrigation with hydrogen peroxide (Sleigh & Linter, 1985). The use of hydrogen peroxide should be restricted to very sloughy wounds, some would also recommend limiting the number of applications or irrigating the wound with saline after use.

Hydrogen peroxide is also available in a stabilized form as a 1.5% cream. In this form the antiseptic action is prolonged.

Iodine

Iodine is a broad-spectrum antiseptic and is available in both an alcohol and an aqueous solution. The aqueous solution is used in wound care, usually as povidone iodine 10% which contains 1% available iodine. It is used as a skin disinfectant and to clean grossly infected wounds. McLure & Gordon (1992) found it to be effective against Methicillin-resistant *Staphylococcus aureus*. Several studies have questioned the value of using povidone iodine. It is cytotoxic to fibroblasts unless diluted to 0.001%, retards epithelialization and lowers the tensile strength of the wound (Lineaweaver *et al.* 1985). Brennan & Leaper (1985) found that povidone iodine 5% damaged the microcirculation of the healing wound, but that a 1% solution was innocuous. Becker (1986) reported that when operating on con-taminated head and neck cases he irrigated 18 with povidone iodine and 17 with isotonic saline. Some 28% of wounds became infected, all of which had been irrigated with povidone iodine.

Some people may have a sensitivity reaction to iodine

The use of povidone iodine should be limited to short-term use on infected wounds where antibiotic therapy is inappropriate.

Povidone iodine is also available in ointment, spray and powder form and impregnated into dressings.

Potassium permanganate 0.01%

This is mostly used on heavily exuding eczematous conditions, mostly associated with leg ulceration. It is mildly deodorizing and has slight disinfectant properties.

It is most easily used in the form of tablets. One tablet dissolved in four litres of water provides a 0.01% solution.

It has been found to cause staining of the skin.

Proflavine

This has a mild bacteriostatic effect on Gram-positive organisms, but not on Gram-negative bacteria. There has been little research to demonstrate its value. Although it is available as a lotion it is mostly used as an aqueous cream. However, the proflavine is not released from the cream into the wound, so has no effect on the bacteria.

Silver nitrate 0.5%

Silver nitrate is rarely used as a lotion. It stains the skin black and prolonged use causes hyponatraemia, hypokalaemia and hypocalcaemia. It is not recommended.

Sodium hypochlorite

Sodium hypochlorite comes in several forms, the commonest being Eusol, Dakin's Solution and Milton.

Sodium hypochlorite was originally used on heavily infected wounds during the First World War. Dakin suggested that for it to be effective, it should be used in large volumes (Thomas, 1990).

Several research studies have been undertaken which suggest that the hypochlorite salts may have little beneficial effect and do much harm. Bloomfield et al. (1985) found the hypochlorite salts cause irritation to both the wound and the surrounding skin, and were found to have a cumulative effect causing redness, pain and oedema and to prolong the inflammatory stage of healing. Sodium hypochlorite is cytotoxic to fibroblasts, unless diluted to a strength of 0.0005%, and retards epithelialization (Lineaweaver et al., 1985). Brennan & Leaper (1985) found that it caused considerable damage to the microcirculation of the wound. The antiseptic effect is lost when it comes in contact with organic material, such as pus or gauze. A study describing the use of Eusol and liquid paraffin on leg ulcers was undertaken by Daltrey & Cunliffe (1981). They found no significant evidence of antibacterial activity. Thomas (1986) found that about 100 ml of Milton were required to dissolve 1 g of yellow slough. He further calculated that, using ribbon gauze 2.5 cm × 1 m soaked in 5 ml of hypochlorite solution, about one hundred dressing changes would be required to remove 5 g of slough (Thomas, 1990).

There seems to be little evidence to show any benefit in using hypochlorites. Now that there is such a wide range of alternative products which can be safely used on sloughy wounds, there seems little or no justification in continuing their use.

2.4.2 Dyes

There are several dyes which have been used to cleanse wounds as they have a mild antimicrobial effect.

Brilliant green

This is infrequently used as a desloughing agent. Little research has been under-taken to study the effect of this solution. However, a study by Niedner & Schopf (1986) found that brilliant green 0.5% significantly retarded granulation. It would seem to be another solution used traditionally with little effort to quantify its value. It is also available combined with lactic acid in gel form.

Crystal violet (Gentian violet)

Gentian violet has been widely used as an astringent. However, it is now only liscenced for use on unbroken skin and as a skin marker. It has been shown to be carcinogenic when used on mucous membranes and open wounds.

Mercurochrome

This is a mercury compound which has bacteriostatic and fungistatic properties. There have been several reports of mercury toxicity following its use, as well as anaphylaxis and aplastic anaemia (Slee *et al.*, 1979; Corrales *et al.*, 1985). There can be no justification for its use.

Lotio rubra or red lotion

This is zinc sulphate lotion. It has to be freshly prepared. It is intended to be applied as a soak. Again, there is little evidence of its benefits or risks and it is rarely used.

2.4.3 Antibiotics

A range of antibiotics is available in topical form. They are potentially hazardous and they are not always absorbed into the wound. There is considerable risk to the patient of sensitization as well as the development of resistant organisms. Systemic antibiotics are the treatment of choice when treating infected wounds because the infection may be too deep for topical antibiotics to penetrate.

D'Arcy (1972) recommends that any antibiotic that is used systemically should not be applied to the skin. However, antibiotics that are not appropriate for systemic use may be developed for use on the skin or in wound care. This means that creams, gels, ointments or impregnated dressings containing gentamycin, tetracycline, fusidic acid or chlortetracycline hydrochloride should not be used as these antibiotics are used systemically. Neomycin is no longer used systemically, but topical use may cause systemic side effects such as ototoxicity. One preparation which would seem to be of benefit in wound care is mupirocin. It has an anti-pseudomonal effect.

2.4.4 Desloughing agents

There are a few desloughing agents which do not fit readily into other categories. These include Miol ®, Aserbine ® and Malatex ®. They have mostly been used on chronic wounds. Little research has been undertaken on these solutions. Extensive use causes maceration of the skin.

2.4.5 Saline 0.9%

This is the only completely safe cleansing agent and is the treatment of choice for use on most wounds. Manufacturers frequently recommend it is used in conjunction with many of the modern wound management products.

2.4.6 Tap water

Tap water is being used more frequently on a variety of wounds. In particular, on areas already colonized, such as wounds following rectal surgery or leg ulcers. Many patients may bath or shower prior to dressing change. There seems to be little point in then 'cleansing' the wound. However, the bath or shower should be thoroughly cleaned afterwards to avoid cross-infection.

2.5 THE OPTIMUM ENVIRONMENT FOR HEALING

In the last few years there has been an explosion in the range of new wound management products available for use. As has already been noted, these dressings have been designed to have a functional effect. The criteria for these products have been defined by Turner (1982) as The 'Optimum Dressing'.

2.5.1 The 'Optimum Dressing'

Turner listed seven criteria for the optimum dressing.

(1) To maintain high humidity at the wound/dressing interface.
(2) To remove excess exudate.
(3) To allow gaseous exchange.
(4) To provide thermal insulation.
(5) To be impermeable to bacteria.
(6) To be free of particles and toxic wound contaminants.
(7) To allow removal without causing trauma to the wound.

Each one of these criteria needs to be considered to examine the underlying research basis.

1. To maintain high humidity at the wound/dressing interface

This criterion is based on the work of George Winter (1962). His research has had a profound effect on wound management. He compared the effect of leaving superficial wounds exposed to form a scab with the effect of applying a vapour-permeable film dressing, using an animal model. Epithelialization was twice as fast in those wounds covered with a film dressing. This was because the dressing maintains humidity on the wound surface. Thus, the epithelial cells were able to slide across the surface of the wound; whereas in the exposed wounds the epithelial cells had to burrow beneath the scab, beneath the dried exudate and beneath the dessicated layers of cells to find a moist layer to allow movement across the wound (see Fig. 2.2).

Later studies have confirmed this finding and identified other benefits as well. May (1984), Alvarez (1987), and Eaglstein (1985) all found local wound pain was considerably reduced in a moist environment, possibly because the nerve endings did not dry out. Studies by Freidman (1983) and Kaufman & Hirshowitz (1983) showed that the moist environment enhanced natural autolytic processes, breaking down necrotic tissue.

(2) To remove excess exudate

Although the wound surface should remain moist, excessive moisture causes maceration of the surrounding skin. The precise balance that needs to be maintained by the dressing between moisture and absorbency is still not certain.

(3) To allow gaseous exchange

Winter & Perrins (1970) found that epithelialization was speeded up when the wound was treated in a hyperbaric oxygen chamber. They concluded that although it was hardly practical to incarcerate patients in hyperbaric oxygen chambers, gaseous exchange on the wound surface was advantageous. However, Knighton *et al.* (1981), found that tissue hypoxia was essential in order to stimulate angiogenesis in the healing wound. A lack of oxygen in the wound creates an area of low oxygen tension, thus stimulating the growth of capillary loops into the wound, bringing oxygen with them. Occlusive dressings which prevent gaseous exchange, such as hydrocolloid dressings, have become widely available and have been seen to be effective. Cherry & Ryan (1985) showed

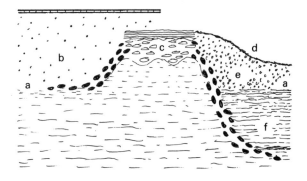

Fig. 2.2 The effect of providing a moist environment for healing: (a) wound surface; (b) moist exudate; (c) epidermis; (d) scab; (e) dry exudate; (f) dry dermis.

that use of an occlusive hydrocolloid dressing stimulated angiogenesis, possibly by maintaining tissue hypoxia.

Silver (1985) concluded that oxygen was essential at all stages of healing, but that the presence of exudate or debris on the wound surface may inhibit gaseous exchange through the dressing. It would be fair to say that the wound does not rely solely on atmospheric oxygen for its oxygen. Whilst the ability of a dressing to allow gaseous exchange may be of benefit at some stages of healing, at others it is either ineffective or unnecessary.

(4) To provide thermal insulation

A constant temperature of 37°C promotes both macrophage and mitotic activity during granulation and epithelialization. Lock (1980) found that there was a significant increase in mitotic activity under dressings that maintained the surface temperature close to core temperature. Cooling of the wound, perhaps by lengthy dressing change, may reduce the surface temperature by several degrees. Myers (1982) studied 420 patients and found that, following wound cleansing, it was 40 minutes before the wound regained its original temperature. Furthermore, he found that it took three hours for mitotic activity to return to its normal rate.

(5) To be impermeable to bacteria

One purpose of a dressing is to provide a barrier between the wound and the environment. The benefits of this are two-fold. First, it prevents contamination of the wound by stopping airborne microorganisms penetrating through to the wound. Second, bacteria on the wound surface are prevented from escaping into the environment and causing cross-infection. However, a soaked or leaking dressing provides a pathway for bacteria in both directions.

(6) To be free of particles and toxic wound contaminants

Many of the older types of dressings, such as gauze tissue or Gamgee shed particles into the wound, particularly open wounds. These particles have been shown to renew or prolong the inflammatory response, affecting the healing rate. Turner (1983) suggested that granulomas may occur and they can damage the strength of the wound, even leading to dehiscence. It should be noted that whilst some of the modern wound management products are made of a particulate matter, such as bead dressings, they do not cause these problems because their construction is quite different.

(7) To allow removal without causing trauma to the wound

There is little point in using a dressing to promote healing, only to find it causes secondary trauma on removal. Damage most frequently occurs when the dressing adheres to the wound surface. This is usually because dried exudate bonds to the dressing, although it may also occur when capillary loops penetrate the dressing.

Removal will cause considerable disruption of newly formed tissue, which delays healing and may lead to a renewed inflammatory response (Turner, 1983).

2.5.2 The nursing implications of the 'Optimum Dressing'

The 'Optimum Dressing' has several implications for nursing practice. They are summarized in Table 2.2. These implications are best discussed by reviewing each criterion.

(1) Maintain high humidity

It should be considered no longer appropriate to use dry dressings on open wounds as a primary dressing. Dry dressings may still be of value as a secondary dressing. When cleaning open wounds, there is no need to dry the wound surface. The skin around the wound should be dried to provide patient comfort and to assist in retaining the new dressing in position.

(2) Remove excess exudate

Depending on the amount of exudate, a secondary pad may be required to provide extra absorbency.

Table 2.2   The 'Optimum Dressing' – nursing implications.

The dressing	Nursing implications
(1) Maintains a high humidity	No dry dressing on open wounds. No need to dry open wounds, just dry skin around wound.
(2) Removes excess exudate	Dressing should have some absorbency. May need to provide a secondary pad.
(3) Allows gaseous exchange	No proven nursing implications.
(4) Thermal insulator	Wounds should not be cleaned with cold lotions. Dressings should not be removed for long periods of time (this also allows wound to dry out).
(5) Impermeable to bacteria	Strapping should be applied like a picture frame. If strike-through occurs either an absorbent pad should be placed on top or the dressing changed.
(6) Free of particles and toxic wound contaminants	Cotton wool should not be used. Any gauze which shreds should not be used. Absorbent pads should not be cut as they will shred.
(7) Removal without trauma	No dry dressings on open wounds. Open wounds should be irrigated in preference to swabbing.

(3) Allow gaseous exchange

As there is still much that is not completely understood in connection with the role of oxygen, there are, as yet, no nursing implications for this criterion.

(4) Thermal insulator

Most dressings provide varying amounts of thermal insulation. It is the use of cold lotions or prolonged dressing change that can have a profound effect on the wound temperature. Therefore, wounds should not be cleaned with cold lotions. The lotion sachet is easily warmed by immersing in hot water. Dressings should not be removed for long periods of time. Not only does this cool the wound, but it allows the wound to dry out and provides an opportunity for contamination by airborne microorganisms.

(5) Impermeable to bacteria

If strapping is used to hold a dressing in place, it should be applied around the edges like a picture frame. Wider strappings are available which may be used to completely cover the wound like an island dressing (see Fig. 2.3). When a dressing soaks through this is known as 'strike-through'. If this occurs, the dressing should be changed as soon as possible. If dressing change is to be delayed for a short time, then the dressing should be covered with an absorbent pad; but, this is only a temporary measure. Many of the modern dressings may leak around the edge,

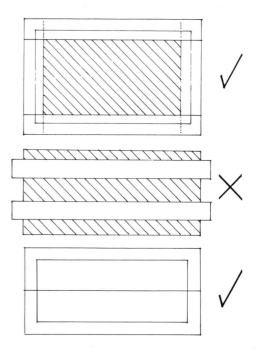

Fig. 2.3   The correct method of applying tape to a dressing.

rather than have strike-through. Once this happens, the life of the dressing cannot be prolonged; it should be changed.

(6) Free of particles

There are many regulations concerning the manufacture of modern dressings, which means that they do not contain particles or contaminants. However, in the UK, cotton wool is still widely used to clean wounds. It is very easy to see the particles it sheds with the naked eye. Therefore, cotton wool should no longer be used to clean wounds. Gauze swabs or irrigation make more appropriate substitutes.

(7) Removal without trauma

The use of dry dressings directly onto the wound surface is the major cause of trauma. This practice should be discontinued. Where practicable, it is better to irrigate a wound rather than swab it because this causes less trauma to the wound during cleaning.

2.5.3 Conclusions

It should be recognized that *no one dressing provides the optimum environment for the healing of all wounds.* Equally, it may be necessary to use more than one type of dressing during the healing of a wound. Many dressings will fulfil some of the criteria and they should be selected following careful assessment of the wound. (See also Chapter 4.)

2.6 MODERN WOUND MANAGEMENT PRODUCTS

In order to make sense of all the dressings that are available, the dressings can be allocated to different categories. They can also be considered in terms of their suitability as a primary or secondary dressing on open wounds.

In the UK, not all the dressings are freely available over the counter in chemists' shops and pharmacies. Government restrictions control which dressings may be prescribed and, in many cases, limit the size range to only a small one. This may considerably affect continuity and quality of care between hospital and home. Changes are taking place gradually, allowing the introduction of some of the newer dressings, but progress is very slow. A particular problem is the very limited choice for the management of cavity wounds.

This section aims to describe the different categories of wound management products and some proprietary examples will be mentioned. A more comprehensive list of proprietary dressings, their usage and application will be found in Appendix A.

2.6.1 Absorbent pads

There are many versions of this type of dressing. Most are in the form of an absorbent core which is covered by a sleeve of gauze or synthetic material. These dressings are not suitable as a primary dressing on open wounds. They do make excellent secondary dressings, however, particularly when there is a heavy exudate.

2.6.2 Adhesive island dressings

These dressings consist of a central pad which is covered with a wider band of adhesive backing. They are light-weight and usually remain in position satisfactorily. There is little absorbent capacity, however. They are widely used on post-surgical wounds which are healing by first intention, but are not suitable as a primary dressing for open wounds.

2.6.3 Alginates

Alginate dressings contain calcium alginate which is derived from seaweed. There are three types of alginate, Kaltostat ®, Sorbsan ®, and Tegagel ®. A further dressing, Fibracol ®, is a variation of alginate also containing collagen. This type of dressing is an interactive dressing because as it reacts with the wound its structure alters. As the dressing absorbs exudate it changes from a fibrous structure to a gel. Sorbsan completely gels, but both Kaltostat and Tegagel maintain their shapes; Fibracol can be removed intact. These dressings are available in a variety of formats, flat dressings, rope or ribbon, extra absorbent versions and with an adhesive backing. They are appropriate for moderate or heavily exuding wounds and may require a secondary dressing. They should not be used on wounds with no or low exudate.

2.6.4 Antibacterials

There are two quite different products in this category. Flammazine ® is a cream containing silver sulphadiazine. It is effective against *Pseudomonas* and *Staphylococcus aureus*. It is widely used on burns. Metrotop ® is a gel containing metronidazole. It reduces odour and anaerobic bacteria and is used on fungating tumours.

2.6.5 Antibiotics

See section 2.4.3.

2.6.6 Antiseptics

See section 2.4.1.

2.6.7 Beads

These dressings are sometimes referred to as dextranomers or xerogels. They are interactive dressings. Several types are available: Debrisan ™, Dermaproof ™, Iodoflex ™ and Iodosorb ™. They consist of powder or beads that swell and gel in the presence of exudate. Various formats have been developed because of the difficulties of application onto relatively shallow wounds. The beads have been incorporated into paste or placed within pads. The powder is also available as an ointment or as a slab of ointment. These products should only be used on moderate to heavily exuding sloughy, necrotic or infected wounds. A secondary dressing is necessary.

2.6.8 Charcoal dressings

These dressings are made from activated charcoal cloth which has been found to be effective in absorbing the chemicals released from malodorous wounds. Infected, necrotic or fungating wounds may have a very unpleasant odour. The dressings come in two types, a charcoal pad, such as Actisorb Plus ™ or Denidor ™, or a combination of dressing and charcoal, such as Carbonet ™, Cliniflex Odour Control ™, Kaltocarb ™ or Lyofoam C ™. The charcoal pad may be used in combination with other dressings. The combination dressing may need a secondary dressing.

2.6.9 Desloughing agents

See Section 2.4.4.

2.6.10 Foams

Foam dressings may be made from polyurethane or silicone. They are available either as a flat foam dressing, such as Allevyn ™, Lyofoam ™ or Tielle ™, or as a filler for cavity wounds, such as Allevyn Cavity Wound Dressing ™ or Silastic Foam ™. They are best used on granulating or epithelializing wounds with some exudate. The management of these dressings varies greatly (see Appendix A). A secondary dressing is not usually needed.

2.6.11 Hydrocolloids

Hydrocolloids are a development from stoma products. They are interactive dressings consisting of a hydrocolloid base made from cellulose, gelatines and pectins, and a backing made from a polyurethane film or foam. As the dressing absorbs exudate it gels to a yellow liquid with a distinctive odour. Unless the nurse or patient is aware that this will occur, it may cause some anxiety. Examples of hydrocolloid dressings include: Biofilm ™, Comfeel ™, Cutinova Hydro ™, Granuflex ™ (known as Duoderm ™ outside UK) and Tegasorb ™. Several come in a wide range of sizes and variations such as more absorbent or thinner than the standard dressing. No secondary dressing is necessary. They can be used on a wide range of wounds, but are most effective on the moderate to low exuding wounds.

2.6.12 Hydrogels

These dressings are made from a co-polymer starch and have a large water content. They come in both thin gel sheets containing 96% water, and as an amorphous gel which is approximately 78% water. The gel sheets such as Gelliperm ™, 2nd Skin ™ or Vigilon ™ are best used on granulating moderate- to low-exuding wounds. The amorphous gel, such as Intrasite Gel ™ may be used on a wider variety of wounds. They require a secondary dressing.

2.6.13 Low-adherent dressings

These types of dressing are low adherent rather than non adherent. They have little if any absorbent capacity and are best on wounds with little exudate. May be used to 'carry' a dressing such as Intrasite Gel ™. They mostly need to be used in combination with an absorbent pad. They do not provide a moist wound environment. Examples of this type of dressing are Melolin ™, NA Dressing ™, Release ™, Silicone-NA ™, Telfa ™ and Tricotex ™.

2.6.14 Low-adherent dressing (medicated)

Inadine ™ is a low-adherent dressing which is impregnated with water soluble povidone iodine. It is suitable for moderate- to low-exuding infected wounds or for prophylaxis in minor traumatic wounds.

2.6.15 Paste bandages

These are cotton bandages impregnated with medicated paste. They are widely used on leg ulcers – particularly when the surrounding skin is eczematous or inflamed. Although they are an effective form of treatment, many patients develop allergies to the contents of the paste. It is wise to patch test the patient before applying a bandage. There are several types of bandage with different pastes such as zinc paste with ichthammol or zinc paste with calamine. A secondary bandage is required.

2.6.16 Sugar paste

Sugar paste has been used in wounds, usually in the form of honey, for many centuries. A more stable paste has been developed using additive-free sugar at Northwick Park Hospital (Middleton & Seal, 1985). It is used on heavily exuding, dirty and malodorous wounds. A secondary dressing is required.

2.6.17 Streptokinase/streptodornase

This is an enzymatic preparation which is presented in the form of powder in a vial. It is reconstituted with normal saline to form a liquid or with a small amount of saline and a lubricating gel to form a jelly. Its action is to debride wounds and it is particularly useful on necrotic eschar. A semipermeable film or gauze may be used as a secondary dressing. Varidase ™ is the only one of this type of dressing available in the UK.

2.6.18 Tulles (non-medicated)

Tulles are also called paraffin gauze, which was originally known as *Tulle Gras*. It is made of open weave cotton or rayon impregnated with soft paraffin. Although the paraffin makes the dressing less adherent, it readily becomes incorporated into granulation tissue: a pattern can be seen on the wound surface when it is removed. It does not maintain a moist wound environment and has no absorbent capacity. It is widely used on minor burns and traumatic injuries. Examples are Jelonet ™, Paranet ™, Paratulle ™ and Unitulle ™. Mepitel ™ has a similar structure but contains silicone gel rather than paraffin. A secondary dressing is required with these dressings.

2.6.19 Tulles (medicated)

Some types of tulles are impregnated with either antiseptics or antibiotics. The commonest type of antiseptic is chlorhexidine and it is present in Bactigras ™, Chlorhexitulle ™ and Serotulle ™. Inadine ™ is slightly different in that it is made of rayon. This dressing is impregnated with povidone iodine ointment. These dressings are useful for superficial infected wounds. Two tulles are impregnated with antibiotics (Fucidin Intertulle ™ and Sofra-Tulle ™). The use of these dressings is not recommended because of the problems of sensitivity and resistance of bacteria.

2.6.20 Vapour-permeable films

There is a wide range of these film dressings available. They provide a moist healing environment but have no absorbency. They should not be used on infected wounds. The method of application varies according to make. Most require a certain amount of skill and practice in application. Examples include Bioclusive ™, Cutifilm ™, Opsite ™ and Tegaderm ™.

2.6.21 Vapour-permeable membranes

An advance on the film dressings are vapour-permeable products which have a certain amount of absorbancy or exudate handling properties. Spyrosorb ™ and Spyroflex ™ are examples of this type of product. They have differing constructions. Products such as Omiderm ™, Surfasoft ™ or Tegapore ™ allow exudate to pass through the dressing and can be left in place for several weeks whilst the outer dressings are changed.

REFERENCES

Alvarez, O.M. & Dellanoy, O.A. (1987) Moist wound healing. Paper presented at American Academy of Dermatology.

Becker,G.D. (1986) Identification and management of the patient at high risk of wound infection. *Head and Neck Surgery*, **8**, 205–210.

Bloomfield,S.F. & Sizer,T.J. (1985) Eusol BPC and other hypochlorite formulations used in hospitals. *Pharmaceutical Journal*, **253**, 153–7.

Brennan, S.S. & Leaper, D.J. (1985) The effect of antiseptics on the healing wound: a study using the rabbit ear chamber. *British Journal of Surgery*, **72**: 10, 780–2.

Brennan,S.S., Foster,M.E. & Leaper,D.J. (1986) Antiseptic toxicity in wounds healing by second intention. *Journal of Hospital Infection*, **8**: 3, 263–7.

Cherry, G.W. & Ryan,T.J. (1985) Enhanced wound angiogenesis with a new hydrocolloid dressing. In Ryan T.J. (ed) *An Environment for Healing: the Role of Occlusion*. Royal Society of Medicine, London.

Corrales Torres, J.L. & De Corres, F. (1985). Anaphylactic hypersensitivity to Mercurochrome (merbrominum). *Annals of Allergy*, **54**, 230–2.

Daltrey, D.C. & Cunliffe, W.J. (1981) A double-blind study of the effects of benzol peroxide 20% and Eusol and liquid paraffin on the microbial flora of leg ulcers. *Acta Dermatology and Venereology*, **61**, 575–7.

D'Arcy,P.F. (1972) Drugs on the skin: a clinical and pharmaceutical problem. *Pharmaceutical Journal*, **209**, 491–2.

Dubranski, S., Duncan, S.E., Harkiss, A., Ball, A. & Robertson, D. (1983) Topical applications in pressure sore therapy. *British Journal of Pharmaceutical Practice*, **5**: 5, 10.

Eaglstein, W,H. (1985) Experiences with biosynthetic dressings. *Journal of the American Academy of Dermatology*, **12**, 434–40.

Forrest, R.D. (1982) Early history of wound treatment. *Journal of the Royal Society of Medicine*, **75**, 198–205.

Freidman, S. & Su, D.W.P. (1983) Hydrocolloid occlusive dressing management of leg ulcers. *Archives of Dermatology*, **120**, 1329–31.

Graber,R.P., Vistnes,L. & Pardoes,R. (1975) The effect of commonly used antiseptics on wound healing. *Plastic and Reconstructive Surgery*, **55**, 272–276.

Johnson, A. (1987) Wound Care, packing cavity wounds. *Nursing Times*, **83**: 36, 59–62.

Kaufman, C. & Hirshowitz, B. (1983) Treatment of chronic leg ulcers with Opsite. *Chirurgica Plastica*, **7**, 211–15.

Kearney, J.N., Arain, T. & Holland, K.T. (1988) Antimicrobial properties of antiseptic impregnated dressings. *Journal of Hospital Infection*, **11**: 1, 68–76.

Knighton, D., Silver, I.A. & Hunt, T.K. (1981) Regulation of wound-healing angiogenesis – effect of oxygen gradients and inspired oxygen concentration. *Surgery*, **90**, 262–70.

Lawrence, J.C. (1987) A century after Gamgee. *Burns*, **13**: 1, 77–79.

Lineaweaver, W., Howard, R., Soucy, D., McMorris, S., Freeman,J., Crain,C., Robertson, J. & Rumley, T (1985) Topical antimicrobial toxicity. *Archives of Surgery*, **120**, March, 267–70.

Lock, P.M. (1980) The effects of temperature on mitotic activity at the edge of experimental wounds. In Lundgren, A. & Soner, A.B. (eds) *Symposia on Wound Healing; Plastic, Surgical and Dermatologic Aspects*. Molndal, Sweden.

May, S.R. (1984) Physiology, immunology and clinical efficacy of an adherent polyurethane wound dressing Opsite. In Wise, D.L. (ed) *Burn Wound Coverings Vol.II*. CRC Press, Boca Raton.

McLure, A.R. & Gordon J. (1992) *In-vitro* evaluation of povidone–iodine and chlorhexidine against methicillin-resistant *Staphylococcus aureus*. *Journal of Hospital Infection*, **21**, 291–9.

Meade, R.H. (1968) *An Introduction to the History of General Surgery*. W.B. Saunders & Co., Philadelphia.

Merchant,J., (1988) Aseptic technique reconsidered. *Care, Science and Practice*, **6**: 3, 74–77.

Middleton, K.R. & Seal, D., (1985) Sugar as an aid to wound healing. *Pharmaceutical Journal*, **235**, 757–8.

Millward, J. (1989) Assessment of wound management in a Care of the Elderly unit. *Care, Science and Practice*, **7**: 2, 47–9.

Murray,Y. (1988) An investigation into the care of wounds in a health authority. *Care Science and Practice*, **6**: 4, 97–102.

Myers, J.A. (1982) Modern plastic surgical dressings, *Health and Social Services Journal*, **92**, 336–7.

Niedner, R. & Schopf, E. (1986) Inhibition of wound healing by antiseptics. *British Journal of Dermatology*, **115**: 31, 41–4.

Reynolds, J.E.F. (ed) (1982) *Martindale: The Extra Pharmacopoeia*. The Pharmaceutical Press, London.

Russell, A.D., Hugo, W.B. & Ayliffe, G.A.J. (1982) *Principles and Practice of Disinfection, Preservation and Sterilisation*. Blackwell Scientific Publications, Oxford.

Silver, I.A. (1985) Oxygen and tissue repair. In Ryan, T.J. (ed) *An Environment for Healing: The Role of Occlusion*. The Royal Society of Medicine, London.

Slee, P.H.Th.J., Ottolander, G.J. & Wolff, F.A. (1979) A case of Merbromin (Mercurochrome ⓉⓂ intoxication, possibly resulting in aplastic anaemia. *Acta Medica Scandinavica*, **205**, 463.

Sleigh, J.W. & Linter, S.P.K. (1985) Hazards of hydrogen peroxide. *British Medical Journal*, **291**, 1706.

Thomlinson, D. (1987) To clean or not to clean. *Nursing Times*, **83**: 9, 71–5.

Thomas, S. (1986) Milton and the treatment of burns. *Pharmaceutical Journal*, **236**, 128–9.

Thomas, S. (1990) Eusol revisited. *Dressing Times*, **3**: 1, 3–4.

Turner, T.D. (1982) Which dressing and why? *Nursing Times*, **78**: 29, suppl. 1–3.

Turner, T.D. (1983) Absorbents and wound dressings. *Nursing*, 2nd series, 12, suppl. 1–5.

Turner, T.D. (1986) Recent advances in wound management products. In Turner,T.D., Schmidt, R.J. & Harding, K.G. (eds) *Advances in Wound Management*. John Wiley & Sons, Chichester.

Walsh, M. & Ford, P. (1989) *Nursing Rituals, Research and Rational Actions*. Heinemann Nursing, Oxford.

Winter, G.D. (1962) Formation of the scab and the rate of epithelialisation of superficial wounds in the skin of the domestic pig. *Nature*, **193**, 293.

Winter, G.D. & Perrins, D.J. (1970) *Proceedings of Fourth International Conference on Hyperbaric Medicine*. Igaku Shoin, Tokyo.

Zimmerman, L.M. & Veith, I. (1961) *Great Ideas in the History of Surgery*. Williams & Wilkins Co., Baltimore.

Chapter 3
The Management of Patients with Wounds

3.1 INTRODUCTION

This chapter looks at assessment of the patient with a wound and how appropriate care may be planned and evaluated. When caring for patients with wounds – of all types – it is important to adopt a holistic approach. There are many factors that can affect the healing process; if they are taken into account when taking a history and assessing the patient it may be possible to mitigate some of the effects. Nursing intervention is not able to resolve *every* problem (e.g. age), but where nursing intervention can be effective, appropriate strategies are suggested.

A model of nursing provides a useful framework for assessing patients. The Activities of Living is the model which has been selected to discuss the factors which can affect healing. However, although this model is very good when considering physical aspects of care, attention must also be given to psychological and spiritual as the three are inextricably linked.

3.2 PHYSICAL CARE

3.2.1 Maintaining a safe environment

Disruption of a safe environment may be responsible for causing wounds, for example, accidents on the road or in the home. Factors within the environment may also affect healing.

Infection

Systemic infection affects healing as the wound has to compete with any infection for white cells and nutrients. Healing may not take place until after the body has dealt with the infection. Systemic infection is frequently associated with pyrexia. Pyrexia causes an increase in the metabolic rate, thus increasing catabolism or tissue breakdown.

All wounds are contaminated with bacteria, especially open wounds. This does not affect healing. However, clinical infection will certainly do so. Infection prolongs the inflammatory stage of healing as the cells combat the large numbers of bacteria. It also appears to inhibit the ability of fibroblasts to produce collagen (Senter & Pringle, 1985).

Infection in a burn wound increases the metabolic rate and thereby increases the time of negative nitrogen balance. Kinney (1977) has shown that there may be a loss of 20-30% of the initial body weight in the presence of major sepsis. Infection also causes pain which raises the metabolic rate (Arturson, 1978).

There have been several major studies of surgical wound infection rates, including Cruse & Foord (1973, 1980), Meers (1981) and Bibby, Collins & Ayliffe (1986). These studies, especially that of Cruse & Foord, have highlighted factors which may predispose the patient to wound infection. It should be noted that the infection rates are usually compared with the expected infection rate of 1.5% for clean surgery. These factors include the following.

Age   It has been found that patients over 65 years are six times more likely to develop an infection in a clean surgical wound than a child under 14 years (Cruse & Foord, 1973). Mishriki *et al*. (1990) found a significantly higher incidence of wound infection in patients over the age of 55 years.

Build/weight for height   Obesity increases clean wound infection rate to 13.5% (Cruse & Foord, 1973). Parrott *et al*. (1989) investigated the reasons for a higher infection rate in emergency Caesarian sections compared with elective surgery: they found obesity to be a significant factor.

Nutritional status   Poor nutrition increases the infection risk. (See also Eating and Drinking 3.24.)

Diabetes   The management of diabetics undergoing surgery must be carefully monitored. Surgery can cause de-stabilization which increases the risk of infection. In turn, infection can also affect the diabetic state. Hyperglycaemia affects the body's defence mechanism by impairing the response of white cells – neutrophils in particular. Cruse & Foord (1973) found a clean wound infection rate of 10.7% in diabetics.

Special risks   Irradiation, steroids, and immunosuppressive drugs cause greatly increased infection rates (Bibby *et al*., 1986.)

Length of preoperative stay   The longer anyone is in hospital, the more chance there is that the patient's skin becomes colonized by bacteria against which the patient has no resistance. Cruse & Foord (1980) found that the clean wound infection rate increased from 1.2% for a 1 day preoperative stay to 2.1% for 7 days and to 3.4% for more than 14 days.

Bed occupancy   Occupancy of more than 25 beds in an open ward increases wound infection (Bibby *et al*., 1986).

Shave   It is impossible to carry out a shave without causing injury to the skin. Bacteria flourish and multiply rapidly in these minute cuts. The clean wound infection rate was found to be 2.5% in shaved patients compared with 1.7% for those who had had their pubic hair clipped and 0.9% for those who were not shaved at all (Cruse & Foord, 1980). Mishriki *et al*. (1990) also found shaving to be a significant factor in the development of infection. They suggest that this is particularly so when contaminated and dirty procedures are undertaken and bacteria are shed on the skin.It is generally recommended that if a patient needs to be shaved preoperatively, it should be done just prior to surgery.

Type of surgery   Infection rates are much higher in some types of surgery than others. This is discussed in more detail in Section 6.2.1. The appearance of infected wounds will be discussed in Section 4.2.6.

The elderly

Elderly people have an increased incidence of underlying disease. Some may directly affect the healing process; others may cause a level of disability which can affect the patient's ability to maintain safe standards of hygiene, thus increasing the risk of infection.

Socioeconomic problems

Poor housing may not only cause hazards such as badly lit stairs, but other problems – damp or rodent infestation, which make it difficult to maintain cleanliness. This predisposes to disease as well as increasing the risk of infection.

● *Nursing assessment* ●

(1) Infection: (a) identify those at risk (see Table 3.1)
            (b) assess wound (see Section 4.2.2)
            (c) monitor temperature regularly.
(2) The elderly: evidence of relevant underlying disease?
(3) Socioeconomic problems: relevant if a chronic wound is to be cared for at home.

● *Nursing interventions* ●

Problem: Actual/potential risk of infection
Goal: Prevention or early detection.

The prevention of infection is the responsibility of all healthcare professionals. There are both general and specific measures which can be taken. Most health authorities have infection control policies which provide guidelines both for the prevention of infection and to reduce the risk of cross infection. The Infection Control Team, especially the Infection Control Nurse can give advice and support.

Much has been written on the prevention of infection. Altemeier *et al.* (1984) provided guidelines on the prevention of infection in surgical patients. They cover such diverse topics as hospital design, housekeeping techniques, the health of the operating personnel, preparation of the patient, methods of sterilization, and more besides. Ayliffe *et al.* (1982) suggested general methods for the management and prevention of hospital-acquired infection, again covering a wide range of topics. Horton (1993) described a strategy for improving the knowledge base of all members of the multidisciplinary team with respect to infection control.

The spread of infection is mostly by people from people. Thus, the simplest and most effective measure to prevent infection is good handwashing. Yet, studies have

Table 3.1   Infection risk factors.

General factors	
Age	Very young or very old.
Nutrition	Emaciated; thin; obese; dehydrated.
Mobility	Limited; immobile; temporary; permanent.
Mental state	Confused; depressed; senile.
Incontinence	Urine; faeces; temporary; permanent.
General health	Weak; debilitated.
General hygiene	Dependence; mouth/teeth; skin.
Local factors	
Oedema	Pulmonary; ascites; effusion.
Ischaemia	Thrombus; embolus; necrosis.
Skin lesions	Trauma; burns; ulceration.
Foreign body	Accidental; planned.
Invasive procedures	
Cannulation	Peripheral; central; parenteral.
Catheterization	Intermittent; closed; drainage; irrigation.
Surgery	Wound; wound drainage; colostomy; implant.
Intubation	Endobronchial suction; ventilation; humidification.
Drugs	
	Cytotoxics; antibiotics; steroids.
Diseases	
	Carcinoma; leukaemia; aplastic anaemia; severe anaemia; diabetes.
	Liver disease; renal disease; transplantation; AIDS.

Based on Bowell, B. (1992).

shown that handwashing is rarely done effectively (Taylor, 1978, Gidley, 1987). Taylor (1978) produced recommendations for handwashing that ensured that all parts of the hands would be washed. Although many nurses are aware of the importance of handwashing, they fail to wash their hands as often as they should (McFarlane, 1990). Guidelines produced by Taylor (1978) identify three different types of handwashing. They include:

Social handwashing   Before the medicine round, before and after eating, when hands are obviously dirty, after going to the toilet and after patient contact.

Antiseptic handwashing   Beginning and end of a shift, before and after aseptic procedures, after handling bedpans and urinals, entering and leaving high risk areas.

Surgical handwashing   Before all surgical procedures.

Gould (1992) has reviewed the studies relating to hand decontamination. She supports the view that hand decontamination is carried out poorly and too seldom. But she also suggests that there has been a failure to consider the reality of the situation in the clinical area. One example cited is that compliance is unlikely if the designated cleanser makes hands sore.

Identification of patients at risk of infection means that appropriate measures can be taken. Some particularly vulnerable patients may require extra measures. These may include the use of a single room with a positive pressure filtered air system, providing protective isolation, prophylactic drugs or special operating techniques, such as a Charnley Howarth tent for orthopaedic procedures.

● *Evaluation* ●

Careful monitoring of vulnerable patients is essential. Monitoring a patient's temperature is a useful means of evaluation as a rise in temperature is often the first indication of infection. The development of clinical audit will identify areas where cross-infection may be a regular problem.

3.2.2 Communicating

The art of communicating is essential to nursing. It involves listening and identifying problems and anxieties as well as giving explanations. Failure to recognize stress or to adequately involve the patient in understanding care can affect wound healing.

Stress and anxiety

Lazerus & Averill (1972) stated that: 'anxiety results when a person is unable to fully comprehend the world around him'. This could be considered in relation to ill health. A further quotation from Frankenhaeuser (1967) adds to this. 'Information is necessary for comprehension, but the perception of this information can be modified by the expectations of the subject'. Many nurses will have seen patients who have not heard or have misunderstood what has been said to them because of their degree of anxiety.

Admission to hospital, whether planned or unplanned, can be a very stressful experience. Stress has a physiological effect. Stimulated by the release of adrenalin, a primary biochemical change in stress is an increased secretion of adrenocorticotrophic hormone (ACTH), which stimulates production of adrenal cortex hormones. In particular, ACTH regulates production of glucocorticoids, cortisol and hydrocortisone. Glucocorticoids cause the breakdown of body stores to glucose, raising the blood sugar. They cause a reduction in the mobility of granulocytes and macrophages, impeding their migration to the wound. In effect, this suppresses the immune system and reduces the inflammatory response. Glucocorticoids also increase protein breakdown and nitrogen excretion which inhibits the regeneration of endothelial cells and delays collagen synthesis. There would seem to be an increased risk of wound infection in a very anxious patient. It has been shown that a reduction of anxiety caused a significant decrease in the incidence of postoperative wound infection (Boore, 1978).

● *Nursing assessment* ●

Zigmond & Snaith (1983) have designed a simple questionnaire which identifies the degree of stress being suffered. It can be filled in by patients (see Fig. 3.1).

HAD Scale

Name: Date:

Doctors are aware that emotions play an important part in most illnesses. If your doctor knows about these feelings he will be able to help you more.
This questionnaire is designed to help your doctor to know how you feel. Read each item and place a firm tick in the box opposite the reply which comes closest to how you have been feeling in the past week.
Don't take too long over your replies: your immediate reaction to each item will probably be more accurate than a long thought-out response.

Tick only one box in each section

I feel tense or 'wound up':
  Most of the time ....
  A lot of the time ....
  Time to time, Occasionally ....
  Not at all ....

I feel as if I am slowed down:
  Nearly all the time ....
  Very often ....
  Sometimes ....
  Not at all ....

I still enjoy the things I used to enjoy:
  Definitely as much ....
  Not quite so much ....
  Only a little ....
  Hardly at all ....

I get a sort of frightened feeling like 'butterflies' in the stomach:
  Not at all ....
  Occasionally ....
  Quite often ....
  Very often ....

I get a sort of frightened feeling as if something awful is about to happen:
  Very definitely and quite badly ....
  Yes, but not too badly ....
  A little, but it doesn't worry me ....
  Not at all ....

I have lost interest in my appearance:
  Definitely ....
  I don't take so much care as I should.....
  I may not take quite as much care ....
  I take just as much care as ever ....

I can laugh and see the funny side of things:
  As much as I always could ....
  Not quite so much now ....
  Definitely not so much now ....
  Not at all ....:...........................

I feel restless as if I have to be on the move:
  Very much indeed ....
  Quite a lot ....
  Not very much ....
  Not at all ....

Worrying thoughts go through my mind:
  A great deal of the time ....
  A lot of the time ....
  From time to time but not too often ..
  Only occasionally ....

I look forward with enjoyment to things:
  As much as ever I did ....
  Rather less than I used to ....
  Definitely less than I used to ....
  Hardly at all ....

I feel cheerful:
  Not at all ....
  Not often ....
  Sometimes ....
  Most of the time ....

I get sudden feelings of panic:
  Very often indeed ....
  Quite often ....
  Not very often ....
  Not at all ....

I can sit at ease and feel relaxed:
  Definitely ....
  Usually ....
  Not often ....
  Not at all ....

I can enjoy a good book or radio or TV programme:
  Often ....
  Sometimes ....
  Not often ....
  Very seldom ....

Do not write below this line

Fig. 3.1 The HAD scale.

Reproduced with permission. Zigmond, A.S. & Snaith, R.P. (1983) *Acta Psychiatrica Scandinavica* (1983) **67**, 361–70.

They found most patients found it simple to use and were enthusiastic about the concept.

● *Nursing interventions* ●

Problem: Anxiety related to hospital admission.
Goal: The patient will be able to express his/her specific anxieties.

Many patients find their admission to hospital a very anxious time. Volicer & Bohannon (1975) found that lack of communication increased stress. The initial assessment, therefore, should provide both information and an opportunity for the patient to ask questions and express his/her feelings and concerns. Not all patients will always be able to discuss their anxieties immediately; it may be a question of an ongoing process of building up a relationship over a period of time. A study by Wilkinson (1992) of cancer patients on six wards in two hospitals showed that most patients desired open communication with those caring for them. Unfortunately, her study found that some nurses blocked communication with patients because they saw it as the doctor's role or they found it too distressing. Others felt that they would like to talk truthfully with their patients, but lacked the skills to do so. Certainly, every nurse should cultivate the art of listening. Morrison & Burnard (1989) suggest that nurses will work more efficiently if they communicate effectively.

Active listening is not a very safe occupation. The consequences may be emotionally painful to the nurse because of the difficult questions that may be asked. Many nurses may feel inadequate or too inexperienced. Koshy (1989) describes active listening as: 'the process of receiving and assimilating ideas and information from verbal and non-verbal messages and responding appropriately'. Tschudin (1991) emphasizes the importance of not making assumptions: it is too easy for a nurse to assume she knows not only the problem, but also has the answers for dealing with it.

Problem: Anxiety related to surgery
Goal: The patient's anxiety will be reduced by adequate pre-operative preparation.

There is now a much greater awareness of the importance of providing good pre-operative information. A Department of Health circular (1990) makes it clear that all patients have the right to understand their treatment and the risks involved. Wilson-Barnett & Fordham (1983) showed that providing an explanation of fears and reassurance promoted recovery. Janis (1958) found that stress levels were as high in patients undergoing what could be classed minor surgery as in those having major surgery. Smith (1992) described how a lack of understanding of the convalescent period following surgery also caused considerable anxiety.

The role of the nurse is to ensure that each patient receives appropriate pre-operative information about the surgery and about what to expect in the post-operative period. Radcliffe (1993) has considered how a suitable strategy can be implemented. She suggests that oral information is reinforced with written leaflets which can be a source of reference to both patients and relatives.

● *Evaluation* ●

Anxiety related to hospital admission: repetition of the assessment will enable the nurse to identify any reduction in stress levels. Anxiety related to surgery: the patient should be able to describe the likely course of events in the perioperative and postoperative periods.

Pain

Pain and anxiety are closely related because pain can increase anxiety and anxiety can increase pain. Blaylock (1968) suggested that this was because the nervous response to pain and to anxiety is the same. Hayward (1975) showed that pre-operative information to reduce anxiety resulted in less postoperative pain. Fear of pain can cause much anxiety to patients.

Several studies have shown that a lack of adequate pain control is common. Sriwatanakul *et al.* (1983) found that postoperative patients were often prescribed inadequate analgesia. Seers (1987) found that nurses did not assess patients' pain adequately and consistently underestimated it. The maxim 'pain is what the patient says it is' is rarely adhered to. Balfour (1989) found that patients suffered unrelieved pain following abdominal surgery, even when analgesia was prescribed. Her study found that 25% of patients experienced severe distress and 37.5% had moderate distress. Yet, of the 16 patients involved, only one received the full amount of prescribed analgesia in the first 24 hours following surgery, and no one at all in the second 24 hour period. A larger study by the Royal College of Surgeons (1990) on pain after surgery found that up to 75% of patients experience moderate to severe postoperative pain. The working party also found that nurses had insufficient commitment to providing adequate pain control and a lack of relevant knowledge. Closs (1992) found that patients' sleep was disturbed by pain. In his study of 100 surgical patients, 49 said the pain was worse at night.

It is not only patients undergoing surgery who experience unrelieved pain. Twycross & Fairfield (1982) found that the majority of patients admitted to a hospice had had pain for more than eight weeks which they described as severe, very severe or excruciating. A more recent study was carried out by Chan *et al.* (1990). They studied the prevalence of chronic pain in diabetics. They found that chronic pain was more common in those suffering from diabetes than in those who did not. Pain was usually reported in lower limbs. They noted that there seemed to be little recognition of the problem or facilities to help resolve it.

Raiman (1986) considered why patients suffered from unrelieved pain. Eight main problem areas were identified. They included low expectation of pain relief from patients, inadequate treatment skills, low treatment aims (i.e. pain is accep-table), inadequate account of pain, inadequate monitoring, poor communication and delays in pain control. As a result of this study a pain observation chart was developed which improved communication between patients and staff and considerably enhanced the quality of pain relief. A review by Baillie (1993) considered the range of pain assessment tools. She found them to have been proven to be successful in clinical practice. However, despite this, they are not widely used. She suggests that it may be due to lack of knowledge or that pain control has a low priority in nursing duties.

A different response to the research into pain relief has been to develop patient-controlled analgesia (PCA). A preliminary study by Clark *et al.* (1989) found that patients receiving PCA were discharged earlier than those receiving conventional analgesia – suggesting that PCA improves physical recovery. They suggest that patient anxiety and perceived intensity of pain may also be reduced. Hunter (1991) describes the use of PCA under the supervision of an acute pain team. The team found that patients required varying doses of morphine over a 24-hour period, ranging from 2 mg to 200 mg. This response to individual need cannot be achieved by an intramuscular regime. Thomas (1993) studied 70 patients receiving PCA and found that 65 had pain relief most of the time. Both patients and staff liked the fact that the patients were in control of their pain relief which, it was found, also reduced the degree of anxiety felt by the patient.

Parsons (1992) gives an overview of studies of cultural aspects of pain and concludes that definitions of pain by both the sufferer and carer are shaped by cultural beliefs. In some cultures free expression of feelings of pain is expected whereas in others it is unacceptable. There needs to be recognition of these cultural differences in order to manage pain successfully.

● *Nursing assessment* ●

A pain chart such as Fig. 3.2 allows a more objective assessment of pain and monitoring of the efficacy of analgesia.

● *Nursing interventions* ●

Problem: Inadequate pain control.
Goal: The patient will be able to express feelings of comfort and relief from pain.

Holzman & Turk (1986) describe pain as a unique experience for each individual. It therefore follows that only the patient can describe its presence and severity. Walsh & Ford (1989) have reviewed many studies looking at the actions and attitudes of nurses towards their patients with pain. They make several recommendations for good practice. These include: asking the patient about his/her pain, using pain charts to monitor the effectiveness of analgesia, and aiming to keep the patient pain-free. Modern systems of drug delivery such as slow-release drugs or intravenous pumps provide constant pain relief that is more effective than the use of injections which have a bolus effect.

An American study, Mennagazzi *et al.* (1991) considered the use of music to reduce pain during minor operations under local anaesthetic. Patients about to undergo suturing of lacerations were randomly selected to either listen to music of their choice, or not. There was a significantly lower score for pain (using a pain chart) in those receiving music diversion than in the control group.

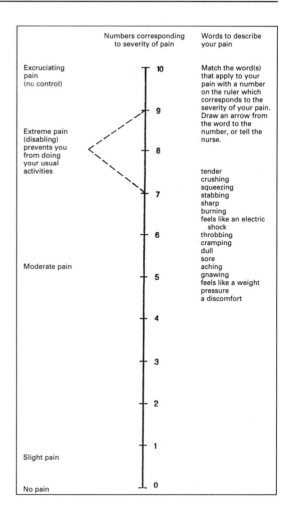

	Numbers corresponding to severity of pain	Words to describe your pain
Excruciating pain (no control)	10	Match the word(s) that apply to your pain with a number on the ruler which corresponds to the severity of your pain. Draw an arrow from the word to the number, or tell the nurse.
	9	
Extreme pain (disabling) prevents you from doing your usual activities	8	
	7	tender crushing squeezing stabbing sharp burning feels like an electric shock
	6	throbbing cramping dull sore
Moderate pain	5	aching gnawing feels like a weight pressure a discomfort
	4	
	3	
	2	
	1	
Slight pain		
No pain	0	

Fig. 3.2 A pain chart.
(From: Bourbonnais, F. (1981).)

Other strategies may be used to assist in pain relief. Measures such as turning, lifting or massage may be very comforting. Simple aids such as a bed cradle to reduce the weight of the bed clothes can be very effective. Distraction therapy – e.g. music – may be of benefit in some circumstances.

● *Evaluation* ●

Regular use of a pain chart allows constant evaluation of the effectiveness of pain relief.

Motivation and education

Stronge (1984) suggests that involving the patient in the care or protection of his wounds promotes healing. Logically, careful explanation of the importance of diet or appropriate exercise can only improve the rate of healing. A positive attitude to healing by the nurse has a significant effect on the outlook of the patient. Fernie & Dornan (1976) found it improved the healing of pressure sores.

The education of surgical patients has been studied extensively in the USA and the UK (Cook,1984). It has been used to reduce the length of hospital admission following surgery and thus costs. A corollary can be drawn: improved recovery implies wound healing without complication.

Another aspect of motivation needs to be considered – that of health beliefs. The concept put forward by Becker (1974) suggests that individuals may recognize the consequences for their health of various actions, but may still be prepared to pay the price for continuing. For example, a patient may know that smoking will increase the risk of having to have a leg amputated, but still not be prepared to give it up. Patient education may have little effect on such an attitude.

Sometimes the patient 'needs' his/her wound. This is not uncommon in patients with leg ulcers. In some regions there is an old wives' tale which says that the ulcer lets the 'bad' out and when the ulcer is healed the person dies. For many housebound people, the only contact with the outside world is with the nurse who comes to dress their leg ulcer. A small study by Wise (1986) followed patients for six months after their leg ulcers were healed. All were assessed for their social contacts. The three patients with the lowest scores had a recurrence of their ulceration. There is obviously an association between social isolation, potential depression and the recurrence of the ulcers.

● *Nursing assessment* ●

Simple questioning can determine the level of relevant knowledge that a patient possesses.

● *Nursing interventions* ●

Problem: A lack of understanding of the care needed to promote wound healing.
Goal: The patient demonstrates the ability to be self-caring and is able to explain his/her plan of care.

In the current climate of early discharge from hospital, many patients will return home with a wound that still requires dressing. If it is practicable, it is helpful to teach the patient to undertake his own dressing. Monitoring and supervision by the district nurse or practice nurse would still be necessary. A planned education programme using short term goals is the most useful. Information about allied care such as diet or exercise can also be incorporated into the programme. Patients with chronic wounds should be given information about their causes and possible prevention.

Some patients will have little motivation to carry on the plan of care once they have been discharged from hospital. Recognition of the reasons for the lack of motivation and good communication with the community staff may be of some help. A few patients will still fail to respond. It is necessary to accept that every patient has the right to choose not to comply with the care recommended by the healthcare team.

● *Evaluation* ●

The ability of the patient to undertake management of the wound will provide adequate evaluation of the effectiveness of the nursing care.

3.2.3 Breathing

A good blood supply to the wound and an adequate supply of oxygen are an essential part of healing. Various factors can adversely affect this.

Age

The circulation is less efficient in the elderly. This may be associated with disease.

Cardiovascular disease

Impaired circulation reduces tissue perfusion. This slows healing and increases the risk of infection. Although tissue hypoxia stimulates angiogenesis (Knighton *et al.*, 1981), it impairs all metabolism and overall growth rate. Peripheral vascular disease is often a complication of diabetes mellitus. It has a detrimental effect on the healing of wounds on the lower limbs and may even be a precipitating factor.

Smoking causes vasoconstriction and is associated with Buerger's disease, a condition causing intermittent claudication and gangrene. Moseley *et al* (1978) suggested that smoking also interfered with the proliferation of erythrocytes, thereby reducing the available oxygen. A review of the effects of smoking on wound healing by Siana *et al.* (1992) found that nicotine affected macrophage activity and reduced epithelialization and wound contraction.

● *Nursing assessment* ●

(1) Cardiovascular disease: previous/present history.
(2) If wound on lower limbs, observe: skin colour
                                          warm/cold legs
                                          presence/absence pedal pulses
                                          oedema.
(3) If known   Hb (normal limits 12–18 g/dl)
               pO_2 (normal limits 11–15 kpa).

3.2.4 Eating and drinking

The activity of eating is essential for health and well-being. It is also essential for wound healing. The particular nutrients that are required have been reviewed by McLaren (1992) and are summarized in Table 3.2. Many studies have considered the importance of nutrition to wound healing. Haydock & Hill (1986) found impaired wound healing in malnourished surgical patients. In a further study (1987) they found that wound healing was improved by giving intravenous nutrition to malnourished surgical patients. Delmi *et al.* (1990) found that malnutrition affected

Table 3.2   The nutrients required for healing.

Nutrient		Contribution
Proteins		Angiogenesis; lymphocyte formation; fibroblast proliferation; collagen synthesis; wound remodelling; immune response; phagocytosis.
Carbohydrates		Provide energy for leucocyte and fibroblast function.
Fats		Formation of new cells.
Vitamins	C	Collagen synthesis; neutrophil function; macrophage migration; synthesis of complement and immunoglobulin; enhances
	A	epithelialization; increases rate of collegen synthesis; improves cross-linking of collagen.
	B complex	Collagen cross-linking.
Minerals	Zinc	Enhances cell proliferation, increases epithelialization, improves collagen strength.
	Manganese Copper Magnesium	Collagen synthesis.

the mortality and morbidity in elderly patients with fractured neck of femur. Warnold & Lundholm (1984) found that malnourished surgical patients were three times more likely to have complications than their well-nourished counterparts. Law *et al.* (1974) found that malnutrition is associated with impaired immunological defence mechanisms, thus increasing the risk of infection. A report from the King's Fund Centre on nutrition (1992) suggests that improved nutrition of hospital patients would reduce the incidence of complications and hospital stay and could save the health service around £266 million each year.

Poor nutrition may be found in those patients suffering from chronic wounds. It may be associated with heavy exudate where protein is being persistantly lost. Mullholland *et al.* (1943) found that one patient with a large pressure sore lost 5.6 g of protein in wound exudate over a 24 hour period. Nylen & Wallenius (1961) found that patients with leg ulcers lost an average of 2.6 g of protein in 24 hours. Malnutrition has also been positively correlated to the development of pressure sores. Pinchkofsky-Devin & Kaminski (1986) assessed elderly patients for nutritional status. All the patients with severe malnutrition had pressure sores. The lower the serum albumin, the more severe was the pressure sore.

Malnutrition is a pathological state which results from a relative or absolute deficiency (or excess) of one or more essential nutrients. As protein or carbohydrates are used in the largest quantities, they are usually the deficient nutrients. This is referred to as protein-energy malnutrition or PEM.

Nutritional status

In her *Notes on Nursing, What it is and What it is Not*, Florence Nightingale said:

'Every careful observer of the sick will agree in this, that thousands of patients are annually starved in the midst of plenty, from want of attention to the ways which alone make it possible for them to take food'. More than a century later this statement is still true. Baughen (1988) reviewed the incidence of hospital malnutrition and found that it is an international problem affecting some 9–65% of patients.

The initial causes of malnutrition may be related to debilitating disease, especially of the gastrointestinal tract, old age, poverty and ignorance. Once admitted to hospital, other factors become relevant. Hamilton Smith (1972) found that patients are starved for up to 12 hours prior to surgery and for varying lengths of time afterwards. Hung (1992) replicated this work and found little change in practice 20 years later. A long period of preoperative starvation serves to compound the effects of trauma and surgery – both of which cause marked catabolism (as discussed in section 3.22). This catabolic state usually lasts between 6 and 18 hours. Following this, the basal metabolic rate rises leading to increased energy requirements. Unless adequate protein and carbohydrate is taken in to supply these needs, further tissue breakdown occurs resulting in muscle wasting and a negative nitrogen balance (see Table 3.3). Lee (1979) suggests that the consequences of a negative nitrogen balance include poor wound healing, impaired immunocompetence and suscept-ibility to infection. Although some patients will return to a normal diet fairly quickly and so redress the balance, others will receive only intravenous fluids. A litre of dextrose 5% contains approximately 150 kilocalories ((kcal) or 'calories'); normal saline does not contain any at all. These fluids obviously do not provide adequate calories to meet the body's requirements.

Burn patients are particularly at risk and may continue to be so for as long as four weeks (Sutherland, 1985). Trauma, burns and pain increase the metabolic rate, further diminishing the patient's nutritional status (Arturson, 1978). Zinc, in particular, is burned up in large amounts during emotional or physical stress. Table 3.4 gives examples of increased energy expenditure following trauma or surgery.

It is the responsibility of the nurse to see that her patients have an adequate diet. Many patients have their mealtimes disrupted by medical ward rounds or being away from the ward undergoing investigations. Older *et al.* (1980) saw food being

Table 3.3 Typical daily postoperative nitrogen loss (g).

Hernia repair	3
Appendicectomy	6
Cholecystectomy	12
Fractured femur	15
Partial gastrectomy	15
Oesophagectomy	90
Peritonitis	18
Sepsis	23

From: Goode, A.W., Howard, J.P. & Woods, S. (1985) *Clinical Nutrition and Diatetics for Nurses.* Hodder & Stoughton, London.
Reproduced by courtesy of the publishers.

Table 3.4 Examples of increased energy expenditure (%).

Elective surgery	24
Skeletal trauma	32
Blunt trauma	37
Trauma with steroids	61
Sepsis	79
Burns	131

N.B. Each 1° rise in temperature increases energy expenditure by 10%

From: Goode, A.W., Howard, J.P. & Woods, S. (1985) *Clinical Nutrition and Dietetics for Nurses*. Hodder & Stoughton, London.
Reproduced by courtesy of the publishers.

placed beyond the reach of a patient and then removed later without the patient ever having the chance to actually eat any of it. Delmi *et al*. (1990) in their study of a group of elderly patients with fractured neck of femur, found that inadequate amounts of food were consumed. It should also be noted that 80% of patients in the study were malnourished on admission. Kirk (1990) found that the food provided in a hospital did not provide all the required nutrients for health in the elderly – particularly vitamins and minerals. Simon (1991) undertook a similar study which showed that the quantities of calories, iron, vitamins C and D, calcium and folic acid provided were inadequate. Although sufficient protein was provided, the patients only ate about 66%. Simon suggested there was a need to supply more nutrient dense food and to review meal times.

Many things can affect the appetite such as anxiety, altered meal times, cultural differences or malaise. It is obvious that a nutritional assessment of all patients should be made on admission and at regular intervals afterwards. Goodinson (1987) has highlighted those patients at risk of developing protein–energy malnutrition (see Table 3.5).

Age

The cell metabolic rate slows with advancing years. There is also an increased risk of malnutrition. Exton Smith (1971) divided the causes into primary and secondary. Primary causes included ignorance, social isolation, physical disability, mental disturbance, iatrogenic disorder and poverty. Secondary causes were impaired appetite, masticatory inefficiency, malabsorption, alcoholism, drugs and increased requirements.

Disease

Diabetes mellitus: uncontrolled glycosuria causes a weak inflammatory response and a reduction in the number of macrophages. Therefore, there is an increased risk of infection and poor healing.

Jaundice: jaundice increases the risk of abdominal dehiscence twelve-fold –

Table 3.5 Conditions increasing risk of malnutrition.

Group/condition	Possible causes/contributing factors
The elderly	Restricted resources for purchasing and storing food, poor dental status, social isolation, depression and bereavement.
Crohns disease Ulcerative colitis	Malabsorption of nutrients; decreased intestinal transit time; diarrhoea.
Gastrointestinal surgery	Protein losses in fistulae and wound exudate. Increased metabolic requirements for protein/energy. Period of postoperative nil by mouth.
Renal, hepatic pancreatic disease	Impose specialist nutrient requirements for protein/energy.
Arthritis	Immobility, inability to manipulate cutlery or prepare food, depression.
Cerebrovascular trauma/ disease, e.g. stroke	Sensory and motor deficits may impair perception of food, taste, smell, mastication, swallowing. Weakness/paralysis, unconsciousness.
Burns, trauma, injury, sepsis	Increased metabolic requirements for protein, energy and micronutrients.
Carcinoma	Taste changes, food aversions, anorexia, nausea, vomiting, diarrhoea may occur as a consequence of the disease and its treatment by chemotherapy/radiotherapy. Carcinoma of the oesophagus, pharynx and gut may constitute mechanical obstruction to intake of food.
Acute and chronic pain	Anorexia; side-effects of analgesic-medications.
Respiratory diseases associated with dyspnoea and hyperventilation	Anorexia and decreased food intake imposed by symptoms. Hyperventilation increases energy requirements.
Medication	Some drugs have catabolic side-effects, e.g. corticosteroids. Nausea, vomiting, diarrhoea due to side-effects of oral drug preparations.
Depression, grief	Anorexia, absence of interest in food.
Obesity	May be overlooked as an 'at risk' group.

From: Goodinson, M. (1987) *Professional Nurse*. **Vol. 2 (11)**, 368.
By courtesy of Austen-Cornish Publishers Ltd.

particularly when associated with malignant disease (Irvin *et al.*, 1978). Taube *et al.* (1981) found that when they added bilirubin to tissue cultures of fibroblasts there were changes in cellular structure and impaired growth of the cells. However, the clinical significance of this is not certain.

Malignant disease: many patients suffering from malignant disease have a reduced nutritional status. Stubbs (1989) found that one in four cancer patients experienced alterations in taste perception which affected their appetite and eating habits.

Drugs

Several drugs affect the nutritional status of patients. Methotrexate has an anti-vitamin effect. This means that the enzyme which would normally bind a vitamin binds the drug instead. Methotrexate competes with folic acid and causes it to be excreted, thereby inhibiting DNA synthesis and cell replication (Holmes, 1987). Neomycin reduces the absorption of vitamins K and D. Para-amino-salicylic acid (PAS) and colchicine reduce the absorption of vitamin B_{12}. A number of drugs can cause a loss of appetite which may lead to a diminished nutritional status. Examples are phenformin, metformin, idomethacin, morphine, digoxin and cancer drugs.

Smoking

Smoking may act as an appetite depressant. Smokers have been found to be deficient in vitamins B_1, B_6, B_{12} and C.

It should also be noted that patients not deemed to be at risk of undernutrition may fail to eat adequately. A study was undertaken by Brown (1991) of patients considered to have no special dietary requirements. She found 68% had intakes of less than 1000 kcal and large deficits of a range of vitamins and minerals. The deficit was caused by failure to eat the food provided. Adequate monitoring of patients' diets is essential.

Charalambous (1993) and her colleagues have devised a nutritional assessment tool which considers various factors which can affect nutritional status. Patients are assessed according to their mental state, diet, ability to swallow, the condition of their mouths and the condition of the skin. The tool provides a score which indicates whether the patient is nutritionally at risk. Such a tool can be helpful in identifying those less obviously at risk of poor nutritional status than those discussed above.

● *Nursing assessment* ●

(1) On admission:
  (a) Identify those at special risk (Table 3.5).
  (b) Take a dietary history.
  (c) Observe for obvious signs of obesity, emaciation or muscle wasting.
  (d) Weigh patient and compare with 'usual weight'. Any % weight change can be calculated with the formula:

$$\frac{\text{usual weight} - \text{current weight}}{\text{current weight}} \times 100$$

  NB this measurement has no value in obesity, fluid retention or dehydration.

  If there is any indication of protein-energy malnutrition (PEM) then the following tests may be used:

(2) Anthropometric measurements: measure skin fold thickness at biceps, triceps, subscapular and suprailiac crest.

The sum of these measurements should be at least 40 cm.

(3) Serum proteins: albumin (normal values 35–50 g/l), it has a half-life of 19 days and so does not change rapidly enough to be an accurate marker, but will indicate chronic PEM;

transferrin (normal values 0.12–0.2 g/l), it has a half life of 9 days and so is a more accurate measure of protein status.

(4) Nitrogen balance: measurement of protein intake and nitrogen output in urine or wound drainage. If output exceeds input then patient is in negative balance.

● *Nursing interventions* ●

Problem: Reduced nutritional status.
Goal: The patient will consume sufficient nutrients for his daily needs.

The nutritional needs for each individual vary according to age, sex, activity and the severity of any illness. If a patient has been assessed as having a reduced nutritional status or falls into a high-risk category, then his nutritional intake should be very carefully monitored. Each patient requires sufficient nutrients to support his basal metabolic rate, his level of activity and the metabolic response to trauma. Patients with heavily exuding wounds, such as fistulae or leg ulcers, may lose large amounts of protein without it being realized.

The hospital dietitian will be able to help in assessing individual needs, so that very specific goals can be set. The goal set at the beginning of this section is of necessity broad, but needs to be more clearly defined for each individual. If a patient is being cared for at home, the carer must also be involved. Many patients will eat better at home, where they can eat what they want, when they want to.

The elderly may have special problems or needs. Penfold & Crowther (1989) have provided helpful guidelines for assisting the elderly to maintain a good diet. One problem may be developing disability. The occupational therapist can give guidance on adapting cooking equipment. Another problem may be lack of education as to what constitutes a 'good' diet. An even simpler problem may be poorly fitting dentures; a new set of teeth may be all that is needed to allow an elderly person to maintain an adequate nutritional status.

For many people, the short period of starvation during surgery followed by a rapid return to an adequate diet will not be harmful and the body will rapidly adapt. However, nurses need to be aware of the amount of food their patients actually eat. These days the plated meal system is widely used in hospitals and there is little monitoring of the amount that patients actually eat. When assisting a patient to plan menus, it is helpful to bear in mind the sources of the nutrients particularly required for wound healing (see Table 3.6).

Some critically ill patients will not have an adequate intake without artificial feeding. This may take the form of a supplement or total nutrition. It can be either by enteral or parenteral feeding. Enteral feeding is the more desirable way of

Table 3.6 Sources of nutrients required for wound healing.

Nutrient		*RDA (adults)	Food source
Protein		42–84 g	Meat, fish, eggs, cheese, pulses, whole-grain cereals.
Carbohydrates		1600–3350 kcals	Wholemeal bread, whole-grain cereals, potatoes, (refined carbohydrates are seen as 'empty' calories).
Vitamins			
	A	750 µg	Carrots, spinach, brocolli, apricots, melon.
	B$_{12}$	3 mg	Meat (especially liver), dairy produce, fish.
	C	30 mg	Fruit and vegetables (but easily lost in cooking).
	D	10 µg	Oily fish, margarine, cod liver oil.
	K		Vegetables, cereals.
Minerals			
	Iron	10–12 mg	Meat (especially offal), eggs, dried fruit.
	Copper		Shellfish, liver, meat, bread.
	Manganese		Tea, nuts, spices, whole cereals.
	Zinc	12–15 mg	Oysters, meat, whole cereals, cheese.

*These are the requirements in health; may need to be increased (see text).

providing nutrition, but if the gastrointestinal tract is not functioning, then total parenteral nutrition is necessary. Holmes (1987) reviewed methods of artificial feeding and provided indications for planning nutritional care.

● *Evaluation* ●

Evaluation may be achieved by regular weighing of the patient and by monitoring serum proteins and nitrogen output.

3.2.5 Eliminating

Uraemia inhibits fibroblast activity, but how this occurs is not yet understood (Lawrence, 1984). McDermott *et al.* (1971) also found that epithelial cell division is depressed. Patients undergoing long-term peritoneal dialysis have a high wound complication following surgery which was seen to be related to poor nutrition and a high urea blood content (Moffat *et al.*, 1982). Barton & Barton (1981) found that a blood urea above 7 mmol/l seriously delayed both granulation and epithelialization.

Incontinence, either urinary or faecal, causes problems of contamination in wounds in the perianal area. They are problematic to dress because of the constant soiling of the dressing.

● *Nursing assessment* ●

(1) Past or present medical history.
(2) Blood urea (normal limits 3.0–6.5 mmol/l)

3.2.6 Personal cleansing and dressing

Poor standards of personal hygiene can affect wound healing because of the increased risk of wound contamination. This may be related to socioeconomic factors (see also Maintaining a safe environment (Section 3.2.1)).

● *Nursing assessment* ●

(1)   Nursing history.
(2)   Observation of personal habits/living accommodation.

3.2.7 Controlling body temperature

Pyrexia may be indicative of infection (see Maintaining a safe environment (Section 3.2.1)). Closs (1985) found a 100% association between perioperative pyrexia and the later development of respiratory infection. However, this finding was not supported in a later study by Payman *et al.* (1989). Pyrexia is a debilitating condition which increases the metabolic rate and is often accompanied by anorexia and dehydration. It may also cause restlessness.

Hypothermia causes a shutdown of the blood supply to the periphery. The blood supply to wounds on the limbs is likely to be severely curtailed. The surface of the wound may become quite necrotic as a result.

● *Nursing assessment* ●

Monitor temperature – 4 hourly – daily, according to the condition of the patient and to the degree of risk of infection.

3.2.8 Mobilizing

People with reduced mobility may have problems with wound healing. Reduced mobility causes stasis in the peripheral circulation, especially in the legs. This often results in stasis oedema and delay in the removal of waste products. Injuries to the legs are slow to heal.

Reduced mobility may also increase the risk of wound development, i.e. pressure sores. This should be taken into account when assessing patients. This topic is explored further in Section 5.2.1.

Drugs

Steroids and rheumatoid drugs have an anti-inflammatory effect. Steroids reduce protein synthesis, capillary budding, fibroblast proliferation and epithelialization (Lawrence,1984). This is probably only of significance in those patients with chronic wounds who are undergoing long-term drug therapy (Lindstrum *et al.*, 1977). Studies have shown that vitamin A will counteract these ill effects (Salmela & Ahonen, 1984).

● *Nursing assessment* ●

(1) Nursing history – degree of mobility.
(2) Physical examination: evidence of oedema, deformity of joints/limbs.
(3) Risk assessment: see Section 5.2.2.

● *Nursing interventions* ●

Problem: Reduced mobility following injury/surgery/illness.
Goal: The patient will regain previous levels of mobility.

Illness from whatever cause can produce feelings of debility. Rest is necessary and a period of time may be spent in bed. As a result of injury or surgery, the patient may find it difficult to move. In most cases the sufferer will regain his previous levels of mobility as he starts to recover. A plan of care should include simple exercises to be undertaken whilst in bed and gradual increases in activity once mobilizing. A series of short term realistic goals may be helpful to both the patient and his nurse. Advice should also be given on the levels of activity to follow after discharge from hospital.

Problem: Reduced mobility due to disability
Goal: The patient will be able to optimize functional mobility

Disability may occur for many reasons and has many levels of severity. Many disabilities result in reduced mobility and immobility is a potential problem. Immobility affects the cardiovascular, respiratory, gastrointestinal, urinary and musculoskeletal systems. The consequences of immobility are far-reaching, as shown by Fig. 3.3. The patient will need to understand these potential problems and how best to avoid them. A multidisciplinary approach is the most effective way of establishing a suitable plan of care for those with major disability. This will ensure that all team members reinforce all aspects of the plan of care. Again, short term goals are the most effective as they provide a sense of achievement as each goal is reached.

Disability does not just gradually disappear. Patients must be prepared for the return to the community. Adaptations to the patient's home may be required. His family or any significant other must be involved in planning and learning to manage any aspects of care that may be needed. Involvement of community-based health professionals must also be established. Appropriate long-term strategies can be established which optimize the patient's abilities whilst preventing potential problems.

● *Evaluation* ●

Continuous evaluation of progress towards goals will enable the constant adaption of goals to realistic levels.

3.2.9 Expressing sexuality

Body image is the mental picture that a person has of him-/herself. Sexuality is an integral part of the image. Body image is also closely associated with self-esteem. Shipes (1987) suggests that self-esteem can be defined as the sum total of all we

IMMOBILITY

Within hours:	**This may lead to:**
venous stasis due to lack of muscular massage;	DVT, pulmonary embolism, skin breakdown;
postural oedema of feet and ankles from sitting with legs down;	intractable stiffness;
stiffness of joints and muscles;	muscular weakness, joint contractures, e.g. dropped foot;
incontinence as unable to get to toilet/ commode;	

After days:	**This may lead to:**
constipation;	faecal impaction;
dehydration due to low fluid intake;	frequency of micturition with oliguria,
pressure sores;	urinary tract infection, septicaemia;
muscular atrophy from disuse;	loss of confidence;
chest infection because of poor ventilation;	pneumonia;
postural hypotension because reflex receptors not activated;	fainting, falls, fractures;
reduced nutritional status due to loss of appetite or poor food;	deficiencies, gastic irritation;

After weeks:	**This may lead to:**
loss of social contact;	depression, purposelessness;
deficiency syndromes, e.g. poor healing, anaemia, loss of bone density;	confusion, heart failure;
weight loss;	contributes to hypothermia if person falls;
loss of ability to care for self;	

Eventually
difficulty in rehabilitating;
further immobility;
death.

Fig. 3.3 The consequences of immobility.

believe about ourselves. All patients with wounds have an altered body image. This can have a profound effect on the person's self-esteem and motivation. Obvious types of wounds which can have these effects are those resulting in disfigurement, such as burns, head and neck surgery, mastectomy, amputation and ostomies. Many patients will also be suffering from anxiety about their prognosis. The resultant stress can be so overwhelming that the patient may be unable to take in information, to share his feelings or to commence rehabilitation. This has physiological effects which delay wound healing (see also Communicating (Section 3.2.2) and Psychological care (Section 3.3)).

● *Nursing assessment* ●

An assessment has been suggested by Shipes (1987). It was developed for ostomy patients, but could also be used for other patients.

(1) Value attached to altered/missing part (could reflect cultural values).
(2) Meaning of altered body to patient.
(3) Support system: family, friends?
(4) Current activities and plans for the future.
(5) Evidence of negative self-esteem? –

       (a) refuses to touch or look at wound?
       (b) refuses to discuss wound?
       (c) verbalizes feelings of worthlessness?
       (d) refuses to participate in care?
       (e) withdraws from social contacts?
       (f) avoids intimate relationships?
       (g) poor grooming?

● *Nursing interventions* ●

Problem: Loss of self-esteem related to altered body image.
Goal: Patient acknowledges change in body image and expresses his/her feelings about this change.

In the early stages, following the circumstances which led to an altered body image, some patients appear to be quite euphoric. This is due to simple relief at having survived. After a while the patient's attitude is likely to change. Common problems that can occur include:

● A sense of loss, similar to bereavement
● Anxiety related to diagnosis, especially if it is cancer
● Loss of sexual function which may be related to type of surgery or trauma or to either of the previous problems
● A withdrawal from social relationships with family or significant others, possibly due to a malodorous wound or any of the previous problems.

The role of the nurse is to assist the patient to develop a re-integrated body image (Shipes, 1987). This may be achieved in a variety of ways. Perhaps the most important is to accept the patient as she/he is, at whatever stage she/he has reached. Allowing a patient to express his feelings and providing him with matter-of-fact information, such as an honest appraisal of the progress of his wound, is beneficial. It is also essential to include family and/or significant others in the patient's care and in any education programme. Good management of the wound should prevent odour or leakage, which will help boost confidence.

As already discussed, under Communication (Section 3.2.2), preoperative information and counselling are most important. Kelly (1989) studied 67 patients who had undergone head-and-neck surgery. Generally, they said they were more anxious before surgery than after. Some 42% of men and 21% of women would have liked more information. Another study by Elspie *et al.* (1989) found that 41%

of patients suffered psychological stress following major surgery for intra-oral cancer.

In many areas, specialist nurses are employed to give help and support to patients, such as stoma nurses or breast care nurses. They can build up a relationship with their patients which give the patient the confidence to express his feelings freely. In other circumstances, it may be a nurse who has a good relationship with a patient who is able to provide this service.

● *Evaluation* ●

Regular evaluation of progress is important for patients with an altered body image. Learning to cope with the new image may take time and strategies may have to be altered along the way. This may be particularly true for those undergoing a series of plastic surgery operations; they may have to cope with a constantly changing body image.

3.2.10 Sleeping

In recent years there has been considerable research on sleep and its effects. Sleep deprivation causes people to become increasingly irritable and irrational (Carter, 1985). They may complain of lassitude and loss of feelings of wellbeing. The sleep–activity cycle is part of the circadian rhythms. During wakefulness the body is in a state of catabolism. Hormones such as catecholamine and cortisol are released. These encourage tissue degradation to provide energy for activity – in particular, protein degradation occurs in muscle. Adam & Oswald (1984) suggest that sleep helps healing. The release of catabolic hormones is inhibited during sleep. Instead, anabolism or tissue repair is promoted by hormones such as somatotrophin, testosterone and prolactin.

There is much evidence that sleep patterns are disturbed in hospital. Hill (1989) suggested that ward routines, such as early morning waking, prevent the patient getting adequate sleep. Also, many patients are disturbed during the night. Walker (1972) found that cardiotomy patients were disturbed approximately 14 times a hour in the immediate postoperative period. Woods (1972) observed a similar group of patients and noted that they were disturbed as many as 56 times during the first postoperative night. Morgan & White (1983) found that intensive care nurses were aware of the importance of sleep, but failed to recognize when they were disturbing their patients unnecessarily.

Other factors may also disturb sleep such as anxiety, pain, being unable to sleep in an accustomed position, uncomfortable beds, noise and a high ambient temperature (Closs, 1990). A further study by Closs (1991) considered in greater detail the extent to which pain disturbed sleep at night. Total night-time sleep was found to be reduced by a mean of one hour compared with normal patterns. Nearly 75% reported that pain had prevented sleep. A mean of 3.3 awakenings during the night was found. Despite the fact that about 50% of patients said that their pain was worse at night, they received less analgesia during this time.

● *Nursing Assessment* ●

(1) Compare 'normal' with present patterns of sleep.
(2) Assess the ward environment – is it conducive to sleeping?
(3) Consider ward routines, do they allow the patient to follow any aspect of usual routines, or are they too rigid?

● *Nursing interventions* ●

Problem: Disruption of normal sleeping patterns.
Goal: The patient is able to sleep a number of hours at night and feels well rested.

Hospitals are not restful places. Many patients joke about going home for a rest. Noise is a major factor which disturbs patients, especially irritating noises. Florence Nightingale (1859) discussed the importance of sleep to the sick. She described some of the noises that disturbed patients. They included rattling keys, creaking shoes and stays (corsets) and the rustle of clothes. Whilst at first glance this may appear quite outmoded, there is still truth in this today. Stead (1985) asked patients what disturbed them at night and found that the major problem was noise, in particular, rattling keys and squeaking shoes. Attention to noise reduction at night is an important aspect of nursing care.

McMahon (1990) suggested four types of sleeplessness:

● Difficulty getting to sleep
● Waking regularly during the night
● Waking early in the morning
● Sleeping for the normal length of time, but not waking refreshed.

Various strategies can be employed to help the patient resolve his specific problems. The provision of a milky drink can be beneficial, especially if the patient normally has one at bedtime. Some people may become hungry after having supper at 5 pm or 6 pm. They may ask their visitors to bring them in a snack. Although there is no evidence that food, in itself, can induce sleep, it is certainly difficult to sleep when hungry. Most people have specific routines that they follow each night. As much as possible this same routine should be followed in hospital. It can introduce a feeling of normality into a strange situation.

Some people find their sleep disrupted because of pain. This may be acute pain following trauma or surgery or a more chronic pain relating to a longstanding illness or condition. Adequate pain control is essential. Pain is a resolvable problem (see also Communicating (Section 3.2.2)). The position of a patient may affect his comfort. It is helpful to ensure that the patient is in a comfortable position, with his bell to hand.

During the night, many fears that are suppressed during the day come to the surface. Sleep may be disturbed because of a particular anxiety. Night-time is a quieter time on the ward. It may provide an opportunity for the nurse to sit and listen to the patient and allow him to express his fears and anxieties. Once this has happened, the patient may be able to return to his normal sleep patterns.

Hospital routines can disrupt normal sleep patterns. The lights of a ward may go off late, around 11 pm and come on again at 6 am (Stead 1985). Patients are woken for their drugs and a drink. It seems not unreasonable for more flexibility to be introduced with a reduction of the 6 am drug round to the minimum and an arrangement not to wake those who would prefer to sleep later.

It should be possible, with careful planning, to provide an environment which is conducive to sleep, and a comfortable patient who is able to benefit from it.

● *Evaluation* ●

Patient questionnaires are a useful way of establishing the success or otherwise of the above plan.

3.2.11 Dying

When caring for terminally ill patients with wounds, there are two factors to consider. First, there may not be adequate time left to the patient for a large wound to heal; second, the disease process may adversely affect the healing process. It is important for these patients that appropriate goals are set for their care. These goals should consider the patient's wishes rather than what the nurse thinks they should be. Patient comfort should be of primary consideration. If the wound cannot be healed, then aggressive treatment should be abandoned and dressings which reduce frequency of dressing change utilized.

● *Nursing assessment* ●

This is not always an easy assessment and other disciplines should be involved.

(1) Identify the problems which distress the patient – e.g. pain at dressing change, heavy exudate, odour.

3.2.12 Medical/other intervention

Cancer chemotherapy

These drugs are used to destroy cancer cells throughout the body, both the primary growth and any metastases. They are most effective on rapidly dividing cells. However, they are unable to differentiate between normal and abnormal cells. The majority of drugs work by destroying DNA, or interfering with protein synthesis or cell division. This directly affects fibroblast synthesis and collagen production. Falcone & Nappi (1984) reviewed the range of drugs available and their effect on surgical wounds. They concluded that chemotherapeutic drugs should not be given perioperatively, but after 7–10 days, when the healing process has become established. A more recent study (Robinson *et al.*, 1990) of the effects of Cisplatin on wound bursting strength supported this view. Administration of the drug preoperatively or one day postoperatively had a detrimental effect which was not seen if Cisplatin was given one week postoperatively.

It should also be remembered that many cancer drugs affect nutritional status by causing nausea and vomiting (see Eating and drinking (Section 3.2.4.)).

Radiotherapy

Radiation effectively destroys cancer cells as they are more radiosensitive than normal cells. A dosage high enough to kill cancer cells does not affect the surrounding cells. However, if the dosage has to be increased there is increased risk of normal tissue necrosing. Luce (1984) describes this as a complication and outlines the relationship between cure and complication. He concludes that, whilst a relatively low cure rate of 42–50% would entail a low incidence of complication, a complication rate of 50% would have to be accepted in order to obtain a cure rate of 80%.

Radiation may affect the healing of an existing wound or it may cause changes to the skin so that any later wound will heal slowly. The skin may show signs of damage from the radiation during treatment. This is known as a radiation reaction and will be discussed in Section 6.5.

Levenson et al. (1984) investigated the use of vitamin A supplements to counteract the effects of radiation on wound healing. In the animal model they found that giving vitamin A supplements was effective. Good results were obtained if the supplementation was started prior to radiotherapy or up to two days after treatment.

● *Nursing assessment* ●

(1)   Check patient history for indications about chemotherapy or radiotherapy.
(2)   History of nausea or vomiting or alteration in eating habits?
(3)   Nutritional assessment (see Eating and drinking (Section 3.2.4)).

3.3 PSYCHOLOGICAL CARE

Nurses have always excelled at the physical care of patients. It is only recently that the emotional needs of patients have been considered. Many situations may cause psychological distress. This may be described as stress. The physiological effects of stress and its effect on wound healing have already been described in the section on Communicating (Section 3.2.2). Factors causing psychological distress may be defined as stressors. Those which may be particularly associated with wounded patients will be discussed in this section. It should be noted that other factors not addressed here may also act as stressors.

Fear

Fear is a common human experience which may be transitory or longer lasting. Illness may release many fears – fear of hospitalization, fear of illness, fear of a life-threatening condition, fear of loss of affection of loved ones, fear of the mutilation of surgery. Such fear creates great stress within the sufferer. This may be made worse by the healthcare team failing to recognize when a patient is experiencing fear and so not allowing him to express his feelings.

Grief

Grief is a normal process which allows adaptation to some major loss in a person's life. The wounded patient may have to come to terms with skin damage from burns, the loss of a limb or breast, or other types of mutilating surgery (see also Expressing sexuality (Section 3.2.9)). Kubler-Ross (1969) described various stages in the grief process. She related them to dying, but they can be applied to all types of grief. The stages are: denial, isolation, anger, bargaining, depression and acceptance (see Table 3.7). Each person will progress through some or all of these stages at a different rate and not necessarily in the same sequence. By listening to the patient and accepting without judgement, the nurse can assist in this process and thus reduce the amount of stress suffered. This may be particularly difficult during the stage of anger as the aggression expressed by the patient is often directed at the main caregivers. Understanding of the cause of the aggression will help the nurse deal with this stage of grief.

Powerlessness

Taylor & Cress (1987) describe powerlessness as: 'the perception of loss of control over what happens to oneself and one's environment'. This is a feeling experienced by many hospital patients as they are placed in the subservient 'patient role'. Even simple decisions such as when to eat or go to bed are taken away from the individual. There is pressure to conform and be a 'good' patient. Stockwell (1972) describes very graphically the fate of the unpopular patient who did not conform to the role the nurses desired from him. A 'good' patient will submit without question to treatment and will not ask too many questions. Although it is to be hoped that nursing has moved forward since 1972, many patients are still aware of their loss of status once they are in hospital. Some may feel depressed because of their feelings of learned helplessness. Others may feel quite euphoric to have survived, which may also be misinterpreted as a lack of compliance.

Table 3.7 The grief process.

Denial   The patient denies the situation by refusing to discuss it or by walking away. This stage can be prolonged by others also denying the problem for the patient.

Isolation   The patient may withdraw within him/herself to start to cope with the situation. He/she may experience feelings of intense loneliness.

Anger   The patient may become very aggressive or critical as he feels very angry that he has been 'chosen' to suffer in this way.

Bargaining   At this stage the patient may try to delay the problem by promising good behaviour.

Depression   Once the patient can no longer deny his problem/illness the feelings of rage and disbelief are gradually replaced by a sense of loss associated with depression. This seems to be a beneficial and constructive emotion.

Acceptance   This is a sense of completion or preparedness for what has or will happen.

Based on Kübler-Ross, E. (1969).

In a society where independence is prized, dependence on others may produce feelings of anger and frustration. Many patients remark that they feel a nuisance because they cannot care for themselves. It may also reduce the feelings of self-worth. An example might be cited of an elderly man with bilateral amputations of his legs. He felt that he had no control of his life and was nothing but a trouble to everyone. Simply being asked to take part in a small research project and then realizing his contribution had been very valuable, greatly raised his self-esteem.

● *Nursing assessment* ●

Although the precise problem may vary, the assessment is the same.

(1) Observe body language: does the patient look relaxed, tense, fidgety, withdrawn; avoid eye contact, hypoactive, hyperactive?
(2) Conversation: does the patient talk excessively, not talk to anyone; ask questions, non-questioning?

Do any of these terms describe the patient:

- angry
- aggressive
- demanding
- anxious
- critical
- depressed
- disorientated

- confused
- confident
- distrustful
- fearful
- passive
- euphoric

● *Nursing interventions* ●

Although nurse training is providing improved knowledge of psychological care, it may be appropriate for the patient to have further help from others, a clinical psychologist, a psychiatric nurse, a chaplain or a trained counsellor.

Problem: Fear due to separation from loved ones or related to unfamiliarity.
Goal: The patient identifies the source(s) of his/her fear and is able to describe his/her feelings.

Once the nurse has been able to recognize that the patient is very frightened, then strategies can be developed to allow the patient the opportunity of expressing his/her specific fears. Time may have to be allowed for 'casual' conversation, especially if the patient has few visitors. Assigning the same nurses to care for the patient can build up confidence. Involving the patient and, possibly, the family in all aspects of planning may be helpful. Patients with any sort of sensory loss will need orientation to the new surroundings.

Problem: Grieving related to loss of or disfigurement to a body part.
Goal: The patient will allow himself to experience the grieving process.

A variety of strategies can be adopted to help the patient move through the grief process. Setting aside time to allow the patient to talk is very important. However, it may be constructive to set time constraints as it can be exhausting for both the patient and the nurse. The patient may prefer to know that he has the undivided attention of the nurse for a set period of time each day, rather than an indeterminate amount of time occasionally. For some individuals, it may be appropriate for others to assist the patient in recognizing and talking through their grief. In those situations, the nurse should be there to support and encourage.

> *Problem: Powerlessness related to feelings of loss of control of the environment.*
> *Goal: The patent will express feelings of having a sense of control and will participate in the planning of care.*

Many healthcare workers fail to recognize the degree to which the 'system' takes charge of the individual once they pass through the doors of a hospital. Whilst in an emergency situation there may be some alteration of priorities, every patient is entitled to be treated with respect. Nurses can play an important role in assisting their patients to remain in control of as many areas of their lives as possible. Patient education not only promotes compliance, but allows the patient to participate in care, thus having a degree of control. Discussing with the patient the times particular treatment should be given and involving him in planning care will reduce feelings of powerlessness.

● *Evaluation* ●

Evaluation of psychological care is not easy. Some indication can be obtained by repeating the assessment and by talking to the patient.

3.4 SPIRITUAL CARE

Spirituality is a concept which many nurses find uncomfortable (Allen, 1991). Spirituality should not just be put into the framework of religion. Everyone, whether they believe in a God or not has spiritual needs. Spirituality can be defined as that within us that responds to the infinite realities of life. Peck (1987) described four sequential stages of spiritual development – chaotic, formal, sceptic and mystic. Whilst some may never progress beyond the first stage, others may do so and then regress during times of emotional stress.

Spiritual needs were identified by Fish & Shelley (1985), as the need for meaning and purpose, the need for love and relatedness and the need for forgiveness. Highfield & Cason (1983) also added the need for hope and creativity. Work by Simsen (1986) gave further insight into each person's need for meaning and purpose in life. A patient will seek to understand why he is suffering in a particular way. Until the patient has found meaning to his disease he cannot cope with what will happen next. Once he has, he can move on to the next stage. Simsen describes it as a continuous pattern – the search for meaning and purpose in life followed by experiencing the meaning which leads to anticipating new meaning. Simsen argues that this can be achieved by the promotion of hope and trust, mediated by good relationships.

If the spiritual needs of individuals are not met, or if they experience a catastrophic event in their lives, the result is spiritual pain or distress. Morrison (1992) discussed spiritual pain and suggested it was the result of the shattering of a person's view of life resulting in a loss of meaning. Spiritual distress is recognized by the North American Nursing Diagnosis Association as a nursing diagnosis. Spiritual distress is defined by Kim *et al.* (1987) as: 'a disruption in the life principle that pervades a person's entire being and that integrates and transcends one's biological nature'. The effect of this is not only on the spirit or the emotions, but also physical. Spiritual distress is a stressor which can affect healing. (See also Communicating (Section 3.2.2) and Psychological care (Section 3.3.))

Spiritual distress can show in a variety of ways. The following are examples of loss of meaning and purpose in life, hopelessness and a need for forgiveness:

- A long-term paraplegic lady found that she was no longer 'in charge' of her large family because of a lengthy stay in hospital. Her purpose and meaning in life had been lost. She became withdrawn and irritable and lost her appetite.
- A patient suffering from multiple sclerosis had become much more disabled and developed pressure sores. She lost all hope in her circumstances and became extremely withdrawn, refusing to be with others and avoiding all eye contact.
- An elderly man, aware that his disease was in its terminal stages became extremely distressed, but would not discuss the reason for this. His son explained that he had not spoken to his brother for 20 years. The man wanted to be forgiven by his brother but did not know how to ask him.

In the context of spiritual distress, acceptance also has significance. A patient may need reassurance that others, particularly family and friends, will accept him/her in the new role as a patient, especially if having to come to terms with a disfiguring wound.

● *Nursing assessment* ●

(1) Does the patient:
   (a) express concern about the meaning of life and death?
   (b) show anger towards God/others?
   (c) question the meaning of suffering/illness/forms of treatment?
   (d) question the value of his own existence and that of others?
   (e) describe inner conflicts about beliefs?
   (f) appear withdrawn and lacking in response?
   (g) show loss of appetite?
   (h) sleep a great deal/not sleep (afraid of not waking)?
   (i) show less interest in treatment and care?

(2) Does the patient make such comments as:
   (a) 'Why is this happening to me?'
   (b) 'I've never done anyone any harm?'
   (c) 'I must have been very wicked to have to suffer all this?'
   (d) 'There's always someone worse off than yourself?'
   (e) 'These things are meant to try us?'

● *Nursing interventions* ●

Problem: Spiritual distress related to separation from religious or cultural ties or from a challenged belief or value system.
Goal: The patient will be able to identify the cause of spiritual distress and specify the assistance required to alleviate it.

Many nurses feel uncomfortable with this type of problem and may seek to avoid or ignore it (Stepnick & Perry, 1992). They may perceive that the only necessary nursing intervention is to arrange for the patient to attend a service in the chapel. Whilst many patients find great comfort from this, spiritual care should be seen in much wider terms. The chaplaincy team can give much support to both the patients and staff by both listening, comforting and counselling when necessary. However, nurses need to have some understanding of the aspects of spiritual care.

There can be no standardized nursing care as there is with postoperative physical care. In this situation, each patient must be cared for in the light of his/her unique needs. Even without strong spiritual beliefs, a nurse can provide spiritual care. Carson (1989) suggests that the most effective way of giving spiritual care is the nurse's offering of self. She goes on to describe this as 'being present so as to touch another's spirit'. Fish & Shelly (1985) list five requirements necessary to be able to achieve this: listening, empathy, vulnerability, humility and commitment.
Listening: This is active listening, giving the patient full attention and noting all the non-verbal as well as verbal cues.
Empathy: This allows the nurse to share the feelings of the patient without losing objectivity. This is essential to enable the patient to consider alternatives.
Vulnerability: As the nurse enters into and shares the patient's feelings, she becomes vulnerable. This may be painful, but can also be rewarding.
Humility: This is not easy, few people want to admit that they do not have the answers in their particular field. A sense of humility will enable the nurse to see that she can learn from her patients. Humility also allows her to accept herself and her patients in all their human frailty.
Commitment: Being with a patient through all the difficult times, sharing the pain as well as the joys, involves considerable commitment.

Evaluation

Just as spiritual assessment is very difficult, so too is evaluation of care. The nurse would hope to see her patient at peace with himself, but that may not be easy to assess. Certainly the patient should no longer exhibit some of the behaviour patterns found in the original assessment.

FURTHER READING

Boore, J.R.P., Champion, R. & Ferguson, M.C. (1987) *Nursing the Physically Ill Adult: A Textbook of Medical-Surgical Nursing.* Churchill Livingstone, London.
Carson, V.B. (1989) *Spiritual Dimensions of Nursing Practice.* W.B. Saunders & Co., Philadelphia.

Gould, D. (1987) *Infection and Patient Care: A Guide for Nurses*. William Heinemann Medical Books, London.

REFERENCES

Adam, K. & Oswald, I. (1984) Sleep helps healing. *British Medical Journal*, **289**, 1400–1.

Allen, C. (1991) The inner light. *Nursing Standard*, **5**: 20, 52–3.

Altemeier, W.A., Burke, J.F., Pruitt, B.A. & Sandusky, W.R. (1984) *Manual on Control of Infection in Surgical Patients*. J.B. Lippincott, Philadelphia.

Arturson, M.G.S. (1978) Metabolic changes following thermal injury. *World Journal of Surgery*, **2**, 203–13.

Ayliffe, G.A., Collins, B.J. & Taylor, L.J. (1982) *Hospital-Acquired Infection, Principles and Prevention*. P.S.G. Wright, Bristol.

Baillie, L. (1993) A review of pain assessment tools. *Nursing Standard*, **7**: 23, 25–9.

Balfour, S.E. (1989) Will I be in pain? Patients' and nurses' attitude to pain after abdominal surgery. *Professional Nurse*, **5**: 1, 28–33.

Barton, A. & Barton, M. (1981) *The Management and Prevention of Pressure Sores*. Faber and Faber, London.

Baughen, R. (1988) Nutrition – the poor relation. *Nursing Standard*, **2**: 43, 24–25.

Becker, M.H. (1974) *The Health Belief Model and Sick Role Behaviour*. Health Education Monographs, Winter.

Bibby, B.A., Collins, B.J. & Ayliffe, G.A.J. (1986) A mathematical model for assessing the risk of post-operative wound infection. *Journal of Hospital Infection*, **8**, 31–9.

Blaylock, J. (1968) Psychological and cultural influences on the reaction to pain. *Nursing Forum*, **7**, 271–2.

Boore, J. (1978) *Prescription for Recovery*. RCN Publications, London.

Bourbonnais, F. (1981) Pain assessment: development of a tool for the nurse and patient. *Journal of Advanced Nursing*, **6**: 4, 277–82.

Bowell, B. (1992) Protecting the patient at risk. *Nursing Times*, **88**: 3, 32–5.

Brown, K. (1991) Improving intakes. *Nursing Times*, **87**: 20, 64–8.

Carson, V. B. (1989) *Spiritual Dimensions in Nursing Practice*. W.B. Saunders & Company, Philadelphia.

Carter, D. (1985) In need of a good night's sleep. *Nursing Times*, **81**: 46, 24-26.

Chan, A.W., Macfarlane, I.A. & Bowsher, D. (1990) Chronic pain in patients with diabetes mellitus: comparison with a non-diabetic population. *Pain Clinic*, **3**: 3, 147–59.

Charalambous, L. (1993) A healthy approach. *Nursing Times*, **89**: 20, 58–60.

Clark, E., Hodsman, N. & Kenny, G. (1989) Improved post-operative recovery with patient-controlled analgesia. *Nursing Times*, **85**: 9, 54–55.

Closs, S.J. (1985) Body composition and post operative hypothermia. Unpublished MPhil Thesis, University of Nottingham.

Closs, S. J. (1990) Influences on patients' sleep on surgical wards. *Surgical Nurse*, **3**: 2, 12–14.

Closs, S.J., (1991) Postoperative pain at night. *Nursing Times*, **87**: 18, 40.

Closs, S.J. (1992) Patients' night time pain, analgesic provision and sleep after surgery. *International Journal of Nursing Studies*, **29**: 4, 381–92.

Cook, T.D. (1984) Major research analysis provides proof patient education does make a difference. *Promoting Health*, **5**: 9, 4–5.

Cruse, P.J.E. & Foord, R., (1973) A five-year prospective study of 23,649 surgical wounds. *Archives of Surgery*, **107**, 206–17.

Cruse, P.J.E. & Foord, R. (1980) The epidemiology of wound infection. *Surgical Clinics of North America*, **60**: 1, 27–40.

Delmi, M., Rapin, C.H. & Bengoa, J.M. (1990) Dietary supplementation in elderly patients with fractured neck of femur. *Lancet*, **235**, 1013–1016.

Department of Health (1990) *Health Service Management – Patient Consent to Examination and Treatment.* Department of Health, NHS Management Executive, London.

Elspie, C.A., Freedlander, E., Campsie, L.M. *et al.* (1989) Psychological distress at follow-up after major surgery for intraoral cancer. *Journal of Psychosomatic Research*, **33**: 4, 441–8.

Exton-Smith, A.N. (1971) Nutrition of the elderly. *British Journal of Hospital Medicine*, **5**, 639–45.

Falcone, R.E. & Nappi, J.F. (1984) Chemotherapy and wound healing. *Surgical Clinics of North America*, **64**: 4, 779–94.

Fernie, Q.R. & Dornan, J. (1976) The problem of clinical trials with new systems for preventing or healing decubiti. In Kenedi, R.M., Dowden, J.M. & Scales, J.T. (eds) *Bedsome Biomechanics.* MacMillan Press, London.

Fish, S. & Shelley, J.A. (1985) *Spiritual Care: the Nurse's Role.* InterVarsity Press, Downers Grove, IL.

Frankenhaeuser, M. (1967) Some aspects of research in physiological psychology. In Levi, L. (ed) *Emotional Stress, Physiological and Psychological Reactions – Medical, Industrial and Military Implications.* Karger, Basle.

Gidley, C. (1987) Now wash your hands. *Nursing Times*, **83**: 29, 41–2.

Goodinson, S.M. (1987) Assessment of nutritional status. *Professional Nurse*, **2**: 11, 367–9.

Gould, D. (1992) Hygienic hand decontamination. *Nursing Standard*, **6**: 32, 33–36.

Hamilton Smith, A. (1972) *Nil by Mouth.* RCN Publications, London.

Haydock, D.A. & Hill, G.L. (1986) Impaired wound healing in surgical patients with varying degrees of malnutrition. *Journal of Enteral and Parenteral Nutrition*, **10**: 6, 550–4.

Haydock, D.A. & Hill, G.L. (1987) Improved wound healing response in surgical patients receiving intravenous nutrition. *British Journal of Surgery*, **74**, 320–3.

Hayward, J. (1975) *Information – a Prescription against Pain.* RCN Publications, London.

Highfield, M.F. & Cason, C. (1983) Spiritual needs of patients: are they recognised?. *Cancer Nursing*, **6**, 187–92.

Hill, J. (1989) A good night's sleep. *Senior Nurse*, **9**: 5, 17–19.

Holmes, S. (1987) Dietetics: artificial feeding. *Nursing Times*, **83**: 31, 49–58.

Holzman, A.D. & Turk, D.C. (1986) *Pain Management.* Pergamon Press, Oxford.

Horton R. (1993) Introducing high quality infection control in a hospital setting. *British Journal of Nursing*, **2**: 15, 746–54.

Hung, P. (1992) Pre-operative fasting. *Nursing Times*, **88**: 48, 57–60.

Hunter, D. (1991) Relief through teamwork. *Nursing Times*, **87**: 17, 35–38.

Irvin, T.T., Vassilakis, J.S., Chattopadhyay, D.K. & Greaney, M.G. (1978) Abdominal healing in jaundiced patients. *British Journal of Surgery*, **65**, 521–2.

Janis, I.L. (1958) *Psychological Stress.* Wiley, New York.

Kelly, R. (1989) *A study of patients who have had surgery in the head and neck region.* Paper given at the RCN Research Scotland Symposium, Nov.

Kim, M.J., McFarland, G.K. & McLane, A.M. (1987) *Pocket Guide to Nursing Diagnoses*, 2nd ed. C.V. Mosby, St Louis.

King's Fund Centre (1992) *A Positive Approach to Nutrition as Treatment.* King's Fund Centre, London.

Kinney, J.M. (1977) The metabolic response to injury. In Richards, J.R. & Kinney, J.M. (eds) *Nutritional Aspects of the Critically Ill*. Churchill-Livingstone, Edinburgh.

Kirk, S.F.L. (1990) Adequacy of meals served and consumed at a long-stay hospital for the elderly. *Care of the Elderly*, **2**: 2, 77–80.

Knighton, D.R., Silver, I.A. & Hunt, T.K., (1981) Regulation of wound healing angiogenesis – effect of oxygen gradients and inspired oxygen concentration. *Surgery*, **90**, 262–70.

Koshy, K.T. (1989) I only have ears for you. *Nursing Times*, **85**: 30, 26–29.

Kubler-Ross, E., (1969) *On Death and Dying*. Macmillan, London.

Lazarus, R.S. & Averill, J.R. (1972) Emotion and cognition with special reference to anxiety. In Spielberger, C.D. (ed) *Anxiety: Current Trends in Theory and Research*. Academic Press, New York.

Law, D.K., Dudrick, S.J. & Abdou, N.I. (1974) The effects of protein calorie malnutrition on immune competence in the surgical patient. *Surgery, Gynaecology and Obstetrics*, **139**, 257.

Lawrence, J.C. & Payne, H.J. (1984) *Wound Healing*. The Update Group, London.

Lee, H.A. (1979) Why enteral nutrition? *Research and Clinical Forums I*, **1**, 15–24.

Levenson, S.M., Gruber, C.A., Rettura, G., Gruber, D.K., Demetriou, A.A. & Seifter, E. (1984) Supplemental Vitamin A prevents acute radiation-induced deficit in wound healing. *Annals of Surgery*, **200**, 494–512.

Luce, E.A. (1984) The irradiated wound. *Surgical Clinics of North America*, **64**: 4, 821–9.

McDermott, F.T., Nauman, J. & De Boer, W.G. (1971) Epithelial cell division in acute renal failure. A radio-autographic study in the oesophagus of the mouse. *British Journal of Surgery*, **58**, 52–55.

McFarlane, A. (1990) Why do we forget to remember handwashing? *Professional Nurse*, **5**: 5, 250–2.

McLaren, S.M.G. (1992) Nutrition and wound healing. *Journal of Wound Care*, **1**: 3, 45–55.

McMahon, R. (1990) Sleep therapies. *Surgical Nursing*, **3**: 5, 17–20.

Meers, P.D. (1981) Report on the National Survey of Infection in Hospitals. *Journal of Hospital Infection*, **2**: 8, 31–39.

Menegazzi, J.J., Paris, P.M., Kersteen, C.H., Flynn, B. & Trautman, D.E. (1991) A randomized controlled trial of the use of music during laceration repair. *Annals of Emergency Medicine*, **20**, 348–50.

Mishriki, S.F., Law, D.J.W. & Jeffery, P.J. (1990) Factors affecting the incidence of post-operative wound infection. *Journal of Hospital Infection*, **16**, 223–30.

Moffat, F.C., Deital, M. & Thompson, D.A. (1982) Abdominal surgery in patients undergoing long-term peritoneal dialysis. *Surgery*, **92**, 598–604.

Morgan, H. & White, B. (1983) Sleep deprivation. *Nursing Mirror*, **157**: 14, Suppl. 8–11.

Morrison, P. & Bernard, P. (1989) Students' and trained nurses' perceptions of their own interpersonal skills: a report and comparison. *Journal of Advanced Nursing*, **14**, 321–9.

Morrison, R. (1992) Diagnosing spiritual pain in patients. *Nursing Standard*, **6**: 25, 36–38.

Moseley, L.H., Finseth, F. & Goody, M. (1978) Nicotine and its effects on wound healing. *Plastic and Reconstructive Surgery*, **92**, 570–5.

Mullholland, J.H., Wright, A.M., Vinci, V. & Shafiroff, B. (1943) Protein metabolism and bedsores. *Annals of Surgery*, **118**, 1015–23.

Nightingale, F. (1859) (repr 1974) *Notes on Nursing, What It Is and What It Is Not*. Blackie & Son, Glasgow and London.

Nylen, B. & Wallenius, G. (1961) Protein loss via exudation from burns and granulating wound surfaces. *Acta Chirurgica Scandinavica*, **122**, 97–100.

Older, M.W.J., Edwards, D. & Dickerson, J.W.T. (1980) A nutrient survey in elderly women with femoral neck fracture. *British Journal of Surgery*, **67**, 884.

Parrott, T., Evans, A.J., Lowes, A. & Dennis, K.J. (1989) Infection following Caesarian section. *Journal of Hospital Infection*, **13**, 349–54.

Parsons, E.P. (1992) Cultural aspects of pain. *Surgical Nurse*, **5**: 2, 14–16.

Payman, B.C., Dampier, S.E. & Hawthorn, P.J. (1989) Postoperative temperature and infection in patients undergoing general surgery. *Journal of Advanced Nursing*, **14**, 198–202.

Peck, M. (1987) *The Different Drum: Community Making and Peace*. Simon & Schuster, New York.

Penfold, P. & Crowther, S. (1989) Causes and management of neglected diet in the elderly. *Care of the Elderly*, **1**: 1, 20–22.

Pinchkofski-Devin, G.D. & Kaminski, M.V. (1986) Correlation of pressure sores and nutritional status. *Journal of American Geriatric Society*, **34**, 435–40.

Radcliffe, S. (1993) Pre-operative information: the role of the ward nurse. *British Journal of Nursing*, **2**: 6, 305–9.

Raiman, J. (1986) Pain relief – a two-way process. *Nursing Times*, **82**: 15, 24–28.

Robinson, S., Falcone, R.E. & Nappi, J.F. (1990) The effect of Cisplatin on wound bursting strength in the rat. *Wounds*, **2**: 3, 116–19.

Royal College of Surgeons of England (1990) *Commission On the Provision of Surgical Services: Report of the Working Party On Pain After Surgery*. Royal College of Surgeons, London.

Salmela, R.J. & Ahanen, J. (1981) The effect of methylprednisalone and vitamin A on wound healing. *Acta Chirurgica Scandinavica*, **147**, 307–11.

Seers, K. (1987) Perceptions of pain. *Nursing Times*, **83**: 48, 37–39.

Senter, H. & Pringle, A. (1985) *How Wounds Heal*. Calmic Medical Division of the Welcome Foundation.

Siana, J.E., Frankild, S. & Gottrup, F. (1992) The effect of smoking on tissue function. *Journal of Wound Care*, **1**: 2, 37–41.

Simon, S. (1991) A survey of the nutritional adequacy of meals served and eaten by patients. *Nursing Practice*, **4**: 2, 7–11.

Simsen, B. (1986) The spiritual dimension. *Nursing Times*, **82**: 48, 41–42.

Shipes, E. (1987) Psycho-social issues, the person with an ostomy. *Nursing Clinics of North America*, **22**: 2, 291–302.

Smith, S. (1992) Tiresome healing. *Nursing Times*, **88**: 36, 24–26.

Sriwatanakul, K., Weis, D.F. & Alloza, J.L. (1983) Analysis of narcotic analgesic use in the treatment of post-operative pain. *Journal of the American Medical Association*, **250**: 7, 926–9.

Stead, W. (1985) One awake, all awake!. *Nursing Mirror*, **160**: 16, 20–21.

Stepnick, A. & Perry, T. (1992) Preventing spiritual distress. *Journal of Psychosocial Nursing*, **30**: 1, 17–24.

Stockwell, F. (1972) *The Unpopular Patient*. Royal College of Nursing, London.

Stronge, J. (1984) Principles of wound care. *Nursing*, **2**: 26, suppl. 7–10.

Stubbs, L. (1989) Taste changes in cancer patients. *Nursing Times*, **85**: 3, 49–50.

Sutherland, A.B. (1985) Nutrition and general factors influencing infection in burns. *Journal of Hospital Infection*, **6**: suppl.B, 31-42.

Taube, M., Elliot, P. & Ellis, H. (1981) Jaundice and wound healing – a tissue culture study. *British Journal of Experimental Pathology*, **62**, 227–31.

Taylor, C.M. & Cress, S.S. (1987) *Nursing Diagnosis Cards.* Springhouse Corporation, Pennsylvania.

Taylor, L.J. (1978) An evaluation of handwashing techniques, parts 1 & 2. *Nursing Times,* **74**: 2; 54 & **74**: 3, 108–110.

Thomas, N. (1993) Patient and staff perceptions of PCA. *Nursing Standard,* **7**: 28, 37–39.

Tschudin, V. (1991) Just four questions. *Nursing Times,* **87**: 39, 46–47.

Twycross, R.G. & Fairfield, S. (1982) Pain in far-advanced cancer. *Pain,* **14**, 303–10.

Volicer, B.J. & Bohannon, M.W. (1975) A hospital stress rating scale, *Nursing Research,* **24**, 352–9.

Walker, B. B. (1972) The postsurgery heart patient: amount of uninterrupted time for sleep and rest during the first, second and third post-operative days in a teaching hospital. *Nursing Research,* **21**: 2, 164–9.

Walsh, M. & Ford, P. (1989) *Nursing Rituals, Research and Rational Actions.* Heinemann Nursing, Oxford.

Warnold, I & Lundholm, K. (1984) Clinical significance of preoperative nutritional status in 215 non-cancer patients. *Annals of Surgery,* **199**: 3, 299–305.

Wilkinson, S. (1992) Good communication in cancer nursing. *Nursing Standard,* **7**: 9, 35–39.

Wilson-Barnett, J. & Fordham, M. (1983) *Recovery from Illness.* John Wiley, Chichester.

Wise, A. (1986) Social ulcers. *Care: Science and Practice,* **4**: 3, 18–23.

Woods, N. (1972) Patterns of sleep in post-cardiotomy patients. *Nursing Research,* **21**, 347–52.

Zigmond, A.S. & Snaith, R.P. (1983) The hospital anxiety and depression scale. *Acta Psychiatrica Scandinavica,* **67**, 361–70.

Chapter 4
General Principles of Wound Management

4.1 INTRODUCTION

This chapter will discuss the general principles of wound management. Specific care of chronic and acute wounds will be considered in later sections. The products mentioned in this chapter have been described in Chapter 2 and so will not be described again. Guidance on the application of the different wound management products can be found in Appendix A.

The ability to make an accurate assessment of a wound is an important nursing skill. It should be carried out in conjunction with an assessment of the patient as discussed in Chapter 3. The aim of the assessment is two-fold: (1) it will provide baseline information of the state of the wound so that progress can be monitored; (2) it will ensure that an appropriate selection of wound management products is made. The management of the different types of wounds will be discussed.

There are several factors to consider when assessing a wound. They are:

(1) The wound classification
(2) The depth of the wound
(3) The shape and size of the wound
(4) The amount of wound exudate
(5) The position of the wound
(6) Wound appearance
(7) The environment of care.

4.2 PLANNING WOUND CARE

4.2.1 Wound classification

Wounds can be classified as chronic, acute and postoperative wounds.
Chronic wounds have been described by Fowler (1990) as being of long duration or frequent recurrence. Typical examples are pressure sores and leg ulcers. The patient may have multifactorial problems which affect his ability to heal his wounds.
Acute wounds are usually traumatic wounds. They may be cuts, abrasions, lacerations, burns or other traumatic wounds. They usually respond rapidly to treatment and heal without complication.
Postoperative wounds are intentional acute wounds. They may be healing by first intention, where the skin edges are held in approximation; sutures, clips or tape may be used. Some surgical wounds are left open to heal by second intention,

usually to allow drainage of infected material. Donor sites are also open wounds.

Whatever the type of wound, the healing process is the same. However, there may be related factors to be considered when managing each of these types of wounds, such as the relief of pressure for pressure sores. The care of chronic wounds will be considered in Chapter 5 and of acute wounds in Chapter 6.

4.2.2 The description of wounds according to depth

This type of classification is widely used in the USA, but generally only used to describe burns or, occasionally, pressure sores in the UK.

Wounds are described in relation to the tissues which are damaged or destroyed. Fig. 4.1 illustrates the different depths of tissue damage.

Erosion is the term used to describe the loss of one or two layers of epithelial cells. There is no depth to this type of wound.

Superficial wounds are wounds where the epidermis has been damaged.

A *partial-thickness wound* is when the epithelium and part of the dermis is destroyed. Hair follicles and sweat glands are only partially damaged. This type of wound is sometimes sub-divided into partial thickness and deep-partial-thickness wounds. When these wounds have a large surface area, hair follicles and sweat glands produce epithelial cells during the stage of epithelialization which form islets of cells on the wound surface, thus speeding the healing process.

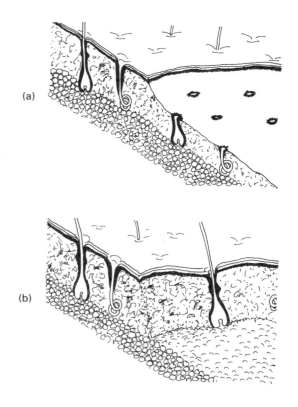

(a)

(b)

Fig. 4.1   The degree of tissue damage in wounds of differing depth. (a) A partial-thickness wound: islands of living epithelium remain around hair shafts and sweat ducts; (b) a full-thickness wound: no living epithelium remains in the injured area.

Full-thickness wounds have all of the epidermis and dermis destroyed. Deeper tissues such as muscle or bone may also be involved. Healing may take longer to establish in these wounds.

4.2.3 Shape and size of the wound

The size and shape of a wound may alter during the healing process (wound measurement is addressed in Section 4.3). In the early stages as necrotic tissue and/or slough are removed, the wound appears to increase in size. This is because the true extent of the wound was masked by the necrotic tissue. Monitoring of wound shape is important to aid in dressing selection – for example, a cavity wound requires a different dressing from a shallow wound; some dressings are not appropriate for use if there is a sinus present. Accurate nursing records are essential for monitoring progress.

4.2.4 The amount of wound exudate

The amount of wound exudate varies during the healing process. There is considerable exudate at the inflammatory stage and very little at epithelialization. A copious exudate may indicate a prolonged inflammatory stage or infection. The amount of exudate also affects dressing selection as a very absorbent dressing may be necessary.

4.2.5 The position of the wound

The position of a wound should be noted as part of the assessment. It may be an indication of potential problems, such as risk of contamination in wounds in the sacral region, or problems of mobility caused by wounds on the foot. Another aspect is the fact that a dressing may stay in place very well on one part of the body but not on another.

4.2.6 Wound appearance

The appearance of the wound gives an indication of the stage of healing that it has reached or of any complication that may be present. Open wounds or wounds healing by second intention can be categorized as:

- Necrotic
- Infected
- Sloughy
- Granulating
- Epithelializing

Some wounds may be seen to have more than one category and so present as 'mixed' wounds. Before assessing a wound, therefore, the nurse should ensure that all the old dressing has been removed. Many modern dressings form a gel which may give a misleading impression of the wound unless it is first cleansed away.

Necrotic wounds (see Plate 1)

When an area of tissue becomes ischaemic for any length of time, it will die. The area may form a necrotic eschar or scab. This can be black or brown in colour. Some necrotic tissue may present as a thick slough which can be brown, grey or off-white. When assessing these wounds it is important to remember that the wound may be more extensive than is apparent. The eschar or slough masks the true size of the wound. Unless the necrotic tissue is removed, the wound will continue to increase in size. Intervention is needed for these wounds to heal.

● *Management* ●

(1) The wound covered with a hard necrotic eschar.
The aim of management is to remove the necrotic tissue from the wound. There are a variety of ways that this can be achieved. If the necrotic tissue is beginning to separate, surgical debridement can be used. This is a very quick way of removing the eschar, but is not always the most appropriate. Wound management products, such as hydrocolloids or an amorphous hydrogel may be used to soften and liquefy the necrotic tissue. It should be noted that as the necrotic tissue liquefies it has a very offensive odour. An enzymatic preparation of streptokinase/streptodornase may also be used, it causes separation of the eschar.
(2) The wound filled with exuding necrotic tissue.
Patients find it very distressing to have a heavily exuding, offensive wound. An alginate dressing may be the most effective when there is heavy exudate. In the case of cavity wounds an alginate rope may be used. If there is a moderate exudate, either hydrocolloids or an amorphous hydrogel can be used. Hydrocolloid powder or paste which can be placed into a cavity and then covered with the hydrocolloid wafer may also be effective. Surgical debridement can be used to remove any loose necrotic tissue. A charcoal dressing can be used to help to reduce odour. It can be used in conjunction with any of the above products, except the hydrocolloids which do not require a secondary dressing.

Infected wounds (see Plate 2)

All wounds are colonized with bacteria. This does not delay healing or mean that wounds will automatically become infected. Cruse & Foord (1980) and Meers (1981) defined an infected wound as one which has a purulent discharge. Other definitions consider the host reaction. If host resistance is adequate to cope with the colonizing bacteria, then no infection will occur. Altemeier (1979) proposed a formula to define this:

$$\frac{\text{Dose of bacteria} \times \text{Virulence}}{\text{Host reaction}} = \text{Probability of infection}$$

Altemeier also suggested local factors that increase the risk of infection:

(1) Devitalized tissue in the wound promotes the colonization of bacteria, especially anaerobes.

(2) Impaired local circulation favours bacterial growth.
(3) Wounds on the abdomen, thigh, calf or buttocks are the most susceptible to infection.
(4) Foreign bodies in a wound can be both irritating and also harbour micro-organisms. This can be true of a sterile suture, even.
(5) Haematomas or 'dead spaces' provide a suitable medium for bacterial growth.

The host reaction to bacterial colonization and the risk of infection has already been discussed in 'Maintaining a Safe Environment' in Chapter 3.

Clinical signs of infection can be observed. They may vary slightly according to the bacteria causing the infection. Usually there is localized erythema or redness. It may be restricted to just one part of the wound, such as at one end of a suture line, or it may spread to a large area around the wound. Associated with the erythema is cellulitis in the adjacent tissues which will also feel hotter than the skin at a distance from the wound. It should be noted that cellulitis is not easy to observe in the presence of oedema. The colour of the exudate and the slough on the wound surface depends on the bacteria causing the infection. There is usually a heavy exudate as the body rushes extra neutrophils and macrophages to the affected area and also tries to 'wash' the bacteria away. The exudate may have an offensive odour and can be the first indication of infection.

● *Management* ●

A wound swab should be taken. This is not to prove that there is infection present as clinical observation has already shown that there is. A swab will assist in identifying the infecting bacteria and then in selecting which are the most appropriate systemic antibiotics. Wound management has to be considered in conjunction with the use of systemic antibiotics.

A variety of products may be used to manage an infected wound. Silver sulphadiazine is especially effective against *Pseudomonas aeruginosa*. Bead dressings may be used. They are especially useful if there is a heavy exudate. Hulkko *et al.* (1981) found Debrisan ™ to be effective on infected wounds. Hillstrom (1988) found Iodosorb ™ reduced the number of bacteria on infected wounds. Alginates are also suitable for infected wounds, but should be changed daily (Thomas, 1990). Some studies, such as Gilchrist & Reed (1988) have suggested that hydrocolloids may reduce the numbers of bacteria on the wound surface. Intrasite Gel ™ may be used on infected wounds (Stewart & Leaper, 1987). However, if there is copious exudate, neither of these two types of dressing will be very effective.

If a wound is infected or potentially infected, but has little exudate, a different strategy may be adopted. Inadine ™, a povidone-iodine tulle, may be used. The iodine is released over varying lengths of time, depending on the amount of exudate. However, no more than four dressings should be applied at any one time.

Sloughy wounds (see Plate 3)

Slough is typically a white/yellow colour. It is most often found as patches on the wound surface, although it may cover large areas of the wound. It is made up of dead cells which have accumulated in the exudate. It can be related to the end of the inflammatory stage in the healing process. Neutrophils have only a short life-span and may die faster than they can be removed. Given the right environment for healing, the macrophages are usually capable of removing the slough and it disappears as healing progresses. Harding (1990) refers to a yellow fibrinous membrane that develops on the surface of some wounds. It is not stuck fast but can be easily removed. The membrane has no effect on healing and recurs if removed. He describes it as a variant on the normal.

● *Management* ●

(1) A shallow sloughy wound with low- to moderate exudate.
The aim of treatment is to promote healing by ensuring that the product used as a primary dressing will provide a moist environment. This will facilitate leucocyte activity. Either hydrocolloids or an amorphous hydrogel will fulfil this requirement.
(2) A shallow sloughy wound with moderate to heavy exudate.
The wound surface should be relatively moist. The dressing should maintain this whilst also controlling the exudate. Several types of products may be used: alginates, beads, hydrocolloids or an amorphous hydrogel.
(3) A cavity, filled with slough and moderate- to low exudate.
The main aim is to assist in liquefying the slough to promote its removal. An amorphous hydrogel or hydrocolloid pastes and wafers may be used. If the slough is very thick, a streptokinase/streptodornase preparation may be used to help to remove it.
(4) A cavity filled with slough and a heavy- to moderate exudate.
These types of wounds sometimes have copious amounts of exudate as the slough liquefies. Initially this may cause concern, but usually granulation tissue will rapidly appear and the amount of exudate will reduce. In these circumstances, alginate rope or ribbon is usually the most effective way of filling the cavity and absorbing the exudate.

When there is less copious exudate a range of dressings can be used, alginate rope or ribbon, beads, amorphous hydrogel or hydrocolloid paste and wafers.

Granulating wounds (see Plate 4)

Granulation tissue was first described by John Hunter in 1786. It relates quite well to the stage of reconstruction in the healing process. The wound colour is red. The tops of the capillary loops cause the surface to look granular, hence the name. It should be remembered that the walls of the capillary loops are very thin and easily damaged, which explains why these wounds bleed easily. Regular, careful measurement will show a reduction in wound volume as the cavity fills with new tissue and contracts inwards.

● *Management* ●

(1) A shallow granulating wound with low- to moderate exudate.
These wounds require very little healing as there is little cavity to fill with granulation

tissue. A moist environment will speed the progress to epithelialization. A range of products may be used: flat foam dressings, hydrocolloids, hydrogels or semi-permeable films.

(2) A shallow granulating wound with moderate- to high exudate.

The amount of exudate is usually less in these wounds than in necrotic, infected or sloughy wounds. The types of dressing that may be used include: alginates, foams, hydrogels and hydrocolloids.

(3) A cavity wound filled with granulation tissue.

The selection of a suitable product depends upon the shape of the cavity and whether there is any undermining or sinuses present. For irregular cavities without sinus formation, a cavity foam dressing such as Silastic Foam ™ may be used, particularly on very large surgical wounds. Other dressings which may be used include alginate rope or ribbon, foam cavity fillers, such as Allevyn ™ cavity wound, hydrogel, Intrasite ™ and hydrocolloid paste and wafers. The selection of these dressings depends on the degree of exudate.

(4) A wound with overgranulation or exuberant granulation tissue.

Occasionally granulation tissue continues to be laid down when a cavity is filled. The granulation tissue stands proud of the rest of the skin. This has been described as exuberant granulation, hypertrophic granulation tissue and also overgranulation. It poses a problem because it prevents epithelial cells from spreading across the wound. Although it has not often been documented, there seems to be a standardized treatment for overgranulation – the use of silver nitrate sticks. They have a caustic effect, thus destroying the proud tissue. Terracortil cream has also been used. No research has been carried out into the use of either of these two products for this purpose. Harris & Rolstad (1993) have investigated an alternative solution of using a flat foam dressing. In a study of 15 wounds they found that the foam dressing significantly reduced the levels of exuberant granulation tissue. This is a much less traumatic method than the use of silver nitrate sticks and can readily be utilized by nurses in any healthcare setting.

Epithelializing (see Plate 5)

As the epithelia at the wound margins start to divide rapidly, the margin becomes slightly raised and has a bluey-pink colour. As the epithelia spread across the wound surface, the margin flattens. The new epithelial tissue is a pinky-white colour. In shallow wounds with a large surface area, islets of epithelialisation may be apparent. The progress of epithelialization may be seen as the new cells are a different colour from those of the surrounding tissue.

● *Management* ●

(1) A shallow epithelializing wound with low- to moderate exudate.

Maintainance of a moist environment and protection of the fragile epithelial tissue are the main aims when choosing a dressing. Suitable dressings include: foams, films, hydrocolloids and hydrogels.

(2) A shallow epithelializing wound with moderate- to heavy exudate.

The aim in treating this type of wound is to control the exudate while also protecting the wound. A variety of dressings can be used: alginates, foams, hydrocolloids and hydrogels.

Care of the skin around the wound

Little attention has been given to the need to care for the skin around a wound. Very often it will be fragile and even malnourished. A range of problems can arise:

(1) Trauma to the skin, particularly from frequent removal of adhesive tapes. Fragile skin may even tear.
(2) Allergy to the tape or dressing, which usually manifests itself as erythema or redness where it was applied. In severe cases there may also be blistering.
(3) Dryness and flakiness of the skin, particularly when bandages are used in conjunction with the dressing. This problem is only likely to occur in chronic wounds where it is not always possible to maintain usual bathing routines. As a result, skin scales are not washed away and collect on the area around the wound.

● *Management* ●

When assessing the wound and planning appropriate care, it is important to assess and monitor the skin around the wound. Little research has been carried out in this area. However, one recent study by Dealey (1992) showed the benefits of using protective skin wipes. Originally developed to be used around stoma sites, skin wipes are widely used in wound care in the USA. Dealey's study showed the benefits of using skin wipes, both to protect fragile skin and when skin trauma and/ or allergy had occurred. Plate 6 shows a patient with severe oedema and fragile skin who had two small ulcerations on her leg. Her skin was protected with a skin wipe and a thin hydrocolloid applied. Plate 7 shows the leg a week later. One ulcer has healed and the skin has remained intact. Plates 8 and 9 show a patient with a superficial pressure sore who had known allergies to film, foam and hydrocolloid dressings. The protective wipe was applied to the skin under a film dressing and the sore was virtually healed within a week. The study demonstrates clearly the benefits of protecting the skin in this way.

Dryness of the skin is more difficult to combat. Emollients can help, but may affect dressing retention. Where it is practicable, bathing or showering using emollients will help to remove skin scales. Creams can also be applied to the affected area avoiding the wound's margins.

There is need for further research into this aspect of wound care.

4.2.7 The environment of care

Consideration must be given to the environment in which care is to be given. Harding (1992) proposed a wound-healing matrix which includes consideration of the environment and carer. The management of a wound can be affected by the circumstances of the patient. For example, the timing of a dressing change may not be very important for a patient in hospital, but for a patient at home, however, perhaps a young mother with children to get to school, timing may be critical. Similarly, flexibility may be important for a patient with a longstanding wound who has to return to work. It may be helpful to arrange for the occupational health nurse in his place of employment to carry out the dressing change, thus reducing the frequency of clinic attendance. Hospital nurses need to ensure that the product selected can be continued after discharge home as not all wound management products are available in the community. Equally, if a non-skilled person is to provide some of the wound care for a patient, then adequate time must be allowed for teaching the individual appropriate routines. Adequate monitoring of care must also be established.

W O U N D   A S S E S S M E N T   F O R M

Name: ....   Date: ....

Position of Wound	Type of Wound
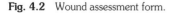	Associated Problems

Wound Appearance   Other Comments

Necrotic	☐	Deep	☐
Clinically infected	☐	Shallow	☐
Sloughy	☐	Offensive	☐
Granulating	☐	Heavy exudute	☐
Epithelialising	☐	Size in cm	.....

Suggested Plan

Fig. 4.2 Wound assessment form.

4.2.8 Evaluating the wound

In order to judge the progress of a wound, it is essential to make objective measurements on initial assessment and to repeat this at regular intervals. Nursing charts can provide a useful framework for this. Fig. 4.2 is an example of an assessment sheet which could be used to record the initial assessment of a wound. Some form of measurement should be incorporated into the assessment. Measurement is discussed in more detail in Section 4.3. Other charts can incorporate ongoing evaluation and are particularly relevant to surgical wounds (see Section 6.2)

If a wound fails to heal or make progress then it is helpful to have a checklist to see if any related factors have been missed. This can be presented in the form of a

Does the patient appear anxious?	→ **YES** →	Encourage patient to express anxieties
↓ **NO** ↓		
Is there oedema or ischaemia around wound site? (especially leg ulcers?)	→ **YES** →	Correct positioning of limbs. Use compression (in oedema); medical opinion
↓ **NO** ↓		
Are there signs of infection – urinary tract, chest, wound?	→ **YES** →	Culture of bacteria, medical opinion; systemic antibiotics
↓ **NO** ↓		
Has patient reduced nutritional status?	→ **YES** →	Cause? Improve nutritional intake
↓ **NO** ↓		
Has patient's general condition deteriorated? (disease-related)	→ **YES** →	Medical opinion
↓ **NO** ↓		
Is patient having sufficient sleep?	→ **NO** →	Cause? Medical opinion? Night sedation or analgesia?
↓ **YES**		

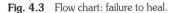

Fig. 4.3 Flow chart: failure to heal.

flow chart such as Fig. 4.3 or as follows:

WOUNDS   Worried, anxious?
                Oedema or ischaemia?
                Urinary tract, chest or wound infection?
                Nutrition poor?
                Disease-related?
                Sleep disturbed?

If this fails to highlight any problem, consider the management of the wound. For example, how long has the dressing been used? It may be up two weeks before an improvement is seen in chronic wounds. Another common problem is the lack of continuity in management: for example, the type of dressing being altered every shift according to the individual whim of the nurse on duty. Rundgren *et al.* (1990) followed the progress of 101 patients with a variety of wounds over a five-month period. They found that from one week to another, about 30% of the patients were receiving a different treatment. Also, that 65% of the wounds did not heal and yet were being treated for the whole of the study period. They concluded that this lack of continuity was related to poor documentation, impatience and a lack of understanding of the healing process.

4.2.9 Evaluating the dressing

Nurses should be prepared to evaluate objectively the dressings they use. This is particularly important if they are using new dressings, although traditional dressings should not be exempt from reappraisal. When evaluating a dressing, various aspects should be considered:

(1) Patient comfort.
(2) Ease of application.
(3) Effectiveness.
(4) Cost.

Patient comfort is of primary importance for any wound management product. It can be very distressing for a patient to suffer painful dressing application. Eusol is well-known for the real discomfort it causes (see Section 2.6.6). Other products may adhere to the wound and cause discomfort to the patient when she/he moves, and when the dressing is removed. A dressing which fails to provide sufficient absorbency and allows leakage of exudate, can cause similar distress as well as considerable inconvenience and feelings of insecurity.

Although different nurses may carry out the dressing, the patient is always the same one! Any evaluation should therefore involve the patient. Many patients like to take an interest and can provide valuable information on new products.

Ease of application means that a dressing can be applied effectively and so stay in place. When using any new product, it may take a little practice to develop the most effective method of application. The nurse should be prepared to try a dressing over a period of time on a variety of wounds (unless contraindicated) and on different parts of the body. This will allow a more comprehensive evaluation. *Effectiveness* is very important. If a product does not promote healing, then it hardly matters whether or not it is comfortable or easy to apply. Before a product becomes available for general use, it should have undergone stringent laboratory tests to check for safety. Marks (1986) also advocates the additional use of models of wound healing. He (rightly) states that it is extremely difficult to conduct good clinical trials on dressing effectiveness as there can be so many variables. Hunt (1983) considered the difficulties of undertaking a clinical nursing trial, and suggested that problems included a lack of control over the admission and discharge of patients, staffing patterns and the large numbers of nurses involved in patient care, and the variations in patterns of care within any health authority.

If nurses are to evaluate the effectiveness of any dressing they use, they need to be aware of any research that has been published. They also need to be able to analyse it critically. Hawthorn (1983) published a checklist giving both guidance in evaluating research reports and advice on undertaking a research project. *Cost* is seen as an important factor in all aspects of care. It should be considered when evaluating any dressing. However, not only the unit cost is relevant; the overall costs should be considered, too. One example is a study by Thomas and Tucker (1989) who compared the use of paraffin tulle with that of an alginate (Sorbsan ™). The results found a reduced overall cost using Sorbsan ™ – despite the fact that the unit cost is greater than that of tulle. All the implications of the cost of healing will be considered in Chapter 8.

4.3 WOUND MEASUREMENT

This section considers the various ways in which a measurement of a wound may be made. Some of them are not really appropriate for use in busy areas, but may have a value in a small scale research study; others are very expensive and outside the pocket of most nurses.

Whatever measurement is used, it should be done on a regular basis, the frequency depending on the type of wound. Chronic wounds should be measured every 2–4 weeks – little change is likely to be seen by more frequent measurement; acute wounds progress much more rapidly, and measurement should be done at each dressing change.

Regular measurement will enable some sort of monitoring of the rate of healing. The final part of this section will look at some of the mathematical methods for measuring the rate of healing, enabling comparison between wounds and different methods of management.

4.3.1 Simple measurement

The very simplest method of measuring a wound is to measure it at its greatest length and breadth and to measure the depth if appropriate. If a wound is a relatively regular shape, such as the example shown in Fig. 4.4, then this can be a fairly successful method. It is also likely to be more accurate if the wound edges are

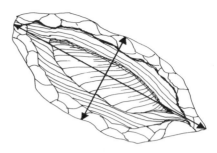

Fig. 4.4 Measurement of a regular-shaped wound.

marked to indicate the measurement points. A probe can be used if the wound is a very irregular shape or has sinus formation.

There are several drawbacks to using this type of measurement. First, the accuracy may be rather doubtful if it is done by many different people.

It is fair to state that even if the same person does the measurement each time, it still may not be measured in the same places or measured accurately. Statistically, this is known as 'sampling error'. Second, if necrotic tissue or slough is present, the true wound size will become apparent as debridement occurs. Wound measurement will show that the wound has increased in size and can give a misleading picture of wound progress. Measurement in this instance will give no indication of wound appearance.

● Overall comment ●

Measurement is best carried out on small, surgically induced cavities, regular in shape and which should heal rapidly. More comprehensive data would be obtained if measurement was used in conjunction with a nursing chart such as that shown in Fig. 4.2.

4.3.2 Wound tracing

Another frequently used system is that of tracing a wound. A variety of materials may be used here, the commonest being acetate paper. One presentation of acetate paper is the lesion measure, samples of which are supplied by several dressing manufacturers. They are usually fairly small sheets with a series of circles on them. The centre circle is 1 cm in diameter and is surrounded by concentric circles which increase in size by 2 cm increments. This gives some estimate of measurement in the tracing.

The surface area of a wound can be calculated quite accurately by placing the tracing over squared paper and counting the number of whole squares. Successive tracings can be compared to show any difference in wound size. If necrotic tissue or slough is present then an initial increase in size will occur as debridement progresses. As with wound measurement, the tracing will show the increase in size without any explanation as it does not provide information on wound appearance or depth. There are also the same risks of inaccuracy. Anthony (1993) describes some of the discrepancies found with this method.

A more sophisticated version of tracing is the use of paper that can be used to convert surface area to weight. A tracing of the wound is made and the shape cut out. This wound shape is then weighed. Likely sampling errors in this method include altering the size/shape of the wound when cutting the paper.

If the acetate sheet is to be placed in direct contact with the wound it will need cleansing with alcohol spray or similar first. Some centres use plastic bags so the underside can be discarded and the side with the tracing retained. Some acetates are provided with disposable backing paper.

● Overall comment ●

Wound tracing is best used on fairly uncomplicated shallow wounds. Ideally, it should be used in combination with an assessment chart, e.g. Figure 4.2.

4.3.3 Photography

The old adage 'a picture is worth a thousand words' may not be strictly true in relation to photographs of wounds, but photography does address some of the criticisms of the previous methods. A photograph provides clear evidence of the appearance of a wound and some suggestion of its size. Myers & Cherry (1984) incorporated a rule in their photographs to provide a scale. Minns & Whittle (1992) describe an aluminium frame attachment to a poloroid camera which has graduated scales to allow calculation of wound size.

When managing chronic wounds, regular photographs can provide real encouragement to both patients and carers.

There are problems, however, with photographs as a record of wound progress. The depth of a wound is not demonstrated in a photograph as it does not accurately record wounds on curved surfaces, and obviously not all nurses have access to a camera (though it may be possible to obtain one on a short-term loan if a dressing trial is being undertaken).

Several factors need to be considered if the purchase of a camera is planned.

● Who will pay for films and developing?
● Is the proposed camera capable of taking close-up pictures?
● Who will be using the camera?
● How can pictures be taken from the same angle and distance each time?
● How can individual patients be identified if using a film with large numbers of exposures?

A Polaroid camera may resolve some of these problems – if a photograph is no good, another can be taken immediately. Whilst the quality may not be as good as more powerful cameras, it is adequate for most needs.

● Overall comment ●

Photographs provide good visual evidence of wound appearance. If a camera is not easily available, photography is best considered only for complicated or unusual wounds. It would be helpful to use some form of wound measurement, such as a scale bar, with the photographs.

4.3.4 Stereophotogrammetry

Stereophotogrammetry is a system which was developed to obtain measurement of the volume of a wound. It does this by providing a three-dimensional picture from two photographs taken simultaneously from different angles. The image thus obtained can be measured. Bulstrode *et al.* (1986) used this method in conjunction with a metrograph and a computer. Goode (1990) considers this method to be far superior to other methods such as tracing or photography. Frantz & Johnson (1992) have developed a method of using stereophotogrammetry with computerized image analysis which they have found to be suitable for clinical trials.

Several drawbacks must be considered. First it is highly unlikely that many nurses would have access to such equipment. Second, special training or the availability of trained personnel would also be necessary. Third it takes about 20 minutes to carry out the procedure. Last, when taking images on a one-off basis, no particular position or point is necessary. However, if a series of pictures is required, the same position should be reproduced each time.

● **Overall comment** ●

Whilst it is interesting to be aware of such equipment, it is not appropriate for everyday use.

4.3.5 Computerized systems of wound measurement

In recent years the development of computer imaging has made dramatic strides. It is used in many ways from providing interior 'views' of a building to giving images of parts of the human body. The potential is enormous. van Riet Paap *et al.* (1991) describe a digital image analysis system made up of a video attached to a computer. The image can be reproduced from the same position each time and can be used on wounds of any size.

A fairly new method involves the use of structured light. Plassmann *et al.* (1993) describe how a camera is connected to an image processing computer which scans the wound which is bathed in light. The computer is able to calculate the wound dimensions. It is unable to measure deep wounds or wounds which change shape.

Another computer program is able to calculate the surface area of a wound. It makes a photocopy of a tracing of the wound from which it makes the necessary calculation. The use of computers is still limited for most nurses. As their use increases, more nurses will become computer literate and confident in using some of the sophisticated programmes available.

● **Overall comment** ●

These are exciting developments, but only available to limited numbers at present.

4.3.6 Measuring the rate of healing

Several researchers have used some of the methods of wound measurement to develop a system for measuring healing. This enables the researcher to compare the healing rate of wounds of different sizes. Although they are not used routinely in many areas, they are of interest.

Gowland-Hopkins & Jamieson (1983) devised a formula to describe the healing rate using wound tracings. The tracings gave information about the original wound circumference, the current wound circumference and the size of the healed area. A formula then calculated the radius of the healed area. Gilman (1990) also proposed a formula based on the linear advance of the wound circumference towards the centre of the wound. He suggested that this could be used on wounds of differing size and would permit an unbiased comparison of the rates of healing.

Resch et al. (1988) put forward a different way of measuring healing rates of pressure sores. They used an alginate compound, commonly used to take dental impressions, to make a mould of a wound. The mould could subsequently be weighed and the volume calculated. The mould also provided a visual record of the shape of the wound. A series of moulds would show the reduction (if any) in size and volume, thus showing the healing rate. They considered that this method was particularly useful on irregularly shaped wounds which are very difficult to measure in other ways.

Marks et al. (1983) observed the rates of healing of 40 laparotomy wounds healing by second intention and 29 pilonidal sinus excisions. The linear regression of healing time against wound size was calculated. Wound size was considered to be the size of the width or depth of the wound, whichever was the greater. A 'predicted' healing time was then calculated for each type of wound. Thus any laparotomy wound or pilonidal sinus excision could be measured and the expected healing time calculated. Early indication of healing problems could then be obtained if the wound failed to maintain the predicted rate of healing. This type of calculation is useful only for regular-shaped surgical wounds which would be expected to heal without complication.

● Overall comment ●

These types of measurement are not likely to be used in general nursing care.

4.3.7 Conclusions

Wound measurement is an important aspect of the assessment and evaluation process. For most wounds, simple operations such as measuring or tracing are quite satisfactory. A series of measurements can be used to give some idea of the rate of healing. It may be useful to use one of the methods of calculating healing rates, if undertaking clinical trials of a specific wound management product. For large-scale studies, access to a computer is usually necessary as manual calculations of large numbers are very time consuming and frequently inaccurate.

REFERENCES

Altemeier, W. A. (1979) Principles in the management of traumatic wounds and in infection control. *Bulletin of New York Academy of Medicine*, **55**: 2, 123–38.

Anthony, D. (1993) The assessment of the skin of the elderly patient with specific reference to decubitus ulcers and incontinence dermatitis. *Journal of Tissue Viability*, **3**: 3, 85–93; 99.

Bulstrode, C.J.K., Goode, A.W. & Scott, P.J. (1986) Stereophotogrammetry for measuring rates of cutaneous healing: a comparison with conventional techniques. *Clinical Science*, **71**, 437–443.

Cruse, P.J.E. & Foord, R. (1980) The epidemiology of wound infection. *Surgical Clinics of North America*, **60**: 1, 27–40.

Dealey, C. (1992) Using protective skin wipes under adhesive tapes. *Journal of Wound Care*, **1**: 2, 19–22.

Fowler, E. (1990) Chronic Wounds: an Overview. In Krasner, D. (ed), *Chronic Wound Care: A Clinical Sourcebook for Healthcare Professionals*, Health Management Publications Inc., King of Prussia, Pennsylvania.

Frantz, R.A. & Johnson, D.A. (1992) Stereophotography and computerised image analysis: a three-dimensional method of measuring wound healing. *Wounds*, **4**: 2, 58–63.

Gilchrist, B. & Reed, C. (1988) The bacteriology of leg ulcers under occlusive dressings. In Ryan, T.J. (ed). *Beyond Occlusion: Wound Care Proceedings*. Royal Society of Medicine, London.

Gilman, T.H. (1990) Parameter for measurement of wound closure. *Wounds*, **2**: 3, 95.

Goode, A.W. (1990) Metabolic basis of wound healing. In Bader, D. (ed) *Pressure Sores – Clinical Practice and Scientific Approach*, Macmillan Press, London.

Gowland-Hopkins, N.F. & Jamieson, C.W. (1983) Antibiotic concentrations in the exudate of venous ulcers: the prediction of the healing rate. *British Journal of Sugery*, **70**, 532–4.

Harding, K.G. (1990) Wound care: putting theory into practice. In Krasner, D (ed). *Chronic Wound Care: A Clinical Sourcebook for Healthcare Professionals*, Health Management Publications Inc., King of Prussia, Pennsylvania.

Harding, K.G. (1992) The wound-healing matrix. *Journal of Wound Care*, **1**: 3, 40–44.

Harris, A. & Rolstad, B.S. (1993) Hypergranulation tissue: a non-traumatic method of management. In Harding K.G., Cherry, G., Dealey, C. & Turner, T.D. (eds.) *Proceedings of the 2nd European Conference on Advances in Wound Management*. Macmillan Magazines Ltd, London.

Hawthorn, P.J. (1983) Principles of research, a check list. *Nursing Times*, **79**: 23, 41–43.

Hillstrom, L. (1988) Iodosorb compared to standard treatment in chronic venous leg ulcers – a multicentre trial. *Acta Chirurgica Scandinavica*, Suppl. 554, 53–56.

Hulkko, A., Holopainen, Y.V.O., Orava, S., Kangas, J., Kuusisto, P., Hyvarinen, E., Ervasti, E. & Silvennoinen, E. (1981) Comparison of dextranomer and streptokinase – streptordinase in the treatment of venous leg ulcers and other infected wounds. *Annales Chirugicae et Gynaecologae*, **70**: 2, 65–70.

Hunt, J. (1983) Product evaluation. *Nursing*, **2**: 12, suppl. 6–7.

Marks, J., Hughes, L.E., Harding K.G., Campbell, H. & Ribeiro, C.D. (1983) Prediction of healing time as an aid to the management of open granulating wounds. *World Journal of Surgery*, **7**: 641–5.

Marks, R. (1986) Assessment of wound dressings. In Turner, T.D., Schmidt, T.D. & Harding, K.G. (eds) *Advances in Wound Management*. John Wiley & Sons, Chichester.

Meers, P.D. (1981) Report on the National Survey of Infection in Hospitals. *Journal of Hospital Infection*, **2**: 8, 31–39.

Minns, J. & Whittle, D. (1992) A simple photographic recording system for pressure sore assessment. *Journal of Tissue Viability*, **2**: 4, 126.

Myers, M.B. & Cherry, G. (1984) Zinc and the healing of chronic leg ulcers. *American Journal of Surgery*, **120**, 77–81.

Plassmann, P., Jones, B.F. & Ring, E.F.J. (1993) Assessment of a non-contact instrument to measure the volume of leg ulcers. In Harding, K.G., Cherry, G., Dealey, C. & Turner, T.D. (eds) *Proceedings of the 2nd European Conference on Advances in Wound Management*. Macmillan Magazines Ltd, London.

Resch, C.S., Kerner, E., Robson, M.C., Heggers, J.P., Scherer, M., Boertman, J.A., & Schileru, R., (1988) Pressure sore volume measurement, a technique to document and record wound healing. *Journal of American Geriatric Society*, **36**, 444–46.

van Riet Paap, E., Mekkes, J.R., Estevez, O. & Westerhof, W. (1991) A new colour video image analysis system for the objective assessment of wound healing in secondary healing ulcers. *Wounds*, **3**: 1, 41.

Rundgren, A., Nordehammar, A., Bjornestol, A, Magnusson, H. & Nelson, C. (1990) Pressure sores in hospitalised geriatric patients. Background factors, treatment, long-term follow-up. *Care – Science and Practice*, **8**: 3, 100–103.

Thomas, S. (1990) *Wound Management and Dressings*. Pharmaceutical Press, London.

Thomas, S. & Tucker, C.A. (1989) Sorbsan in the management of leg ulcers. *Pharmaceutical Journal*, **243**, 706–709

Chapter 5
The Management of Patients with Chronic Wounds

5.1 INTRODUCTION

A chronic wound was defined by Fowler (1990) as one where there is tissue deficit as the result of longstanding injury or insult or frequent recurrence. Despite medical or nursing care these wounds do not heal easily. They are more likely to occur in the elderly or those with multisystem problems. This section will consider the care of patients with pressure sores, leg ulcers and fungating wounds.

Chronic wounds cause much discomfort and pain. A multidisciplinary approach is needed for their management and prevention. Nurses can play an important role in the team as they will usually have the most contact with the patient. An essential part of this role is communication and co-operation across the disciplines. Healing is not possible for all chronic wounds and in these cases the goal is to assist the patient to achieve the maximum independence and function possible.

5.2 THE PREVENTION AND MANAGEMENT OF PRESSURE SORES

Pressure sores are also called 'pressure ulcers', 'bed sores' and 'decubitus ulcers'. A pressure sore can be described as localized damage to the skin caused by disruption of the blood supply to the area, usually caused by pressure, shear or friction, or a combination of any of these. Pressure sores have been known of for centuries. The prophet Isaiah who lived in the eighth century BC, referred to Israel as being covered in bruises and sores and open wounds. Krasner (1990) has reviewed the theories in relation to pressure sores over the centuries.

For many years pressure sores were seen as a failure of care, in particular, the result of bad nursing. Florence Nightingale (1861) saw pressure sores as the fault of the nurse rather than the disease. A famous French doctor, Charcot, believed that doctors could do nothing about pressure sores. As a result, pressure sores became a very emotive issue and were only discussed by doctors as 'A nursing problem' and by nurses with comments like 'We do not have pressure sores here'.

This attitude is now changing and there is greater awareness that rather than cast blame on someone else, the actual cause for a pressure sore should be found. However, nurses still have responsibilities in relation to pressure sores. Dealey (1989a) suggested that nursing responsibilities should include: up-to-date practice, acting as a co-ordinator of care involving other healthcare professionals, facilitating appropriate use of equipment, as an educator and policy-maker and being involved in research.

5.2.1 The aetiology of pressure sores

Pressure sores are caused by a combination of factors both outside and inside the patient.

External factors

There are three external factors that can cause pressure sores either on their own or in any combination of the three. They are pressure, shear and friction.

Pressure is the most important factor in pressure sore development. When the soft tissue of the body is compressed between a bony prominence and a hard surface causing pressures greater than capillary pressure, localized ischaemia occurs. The normal body response to such pressure is to shift position so that the pressure is redistributed. When pressure is relieved a red area appears over the bony prominence. This is called reactive hyperaemia and is the result of a temporarily increased blood supply to the area, removing waste products and bringing oxygen and nutrients. It is a normal body response.

Capillary pressure is generally described as being approximately 32 mmHg, based on the research of Landis (1931). His research was carried out on young, healthy students. He found the average arteriolar pressure was 32 mmHg, but the average pressure in the venules was 12 mmHg. There is also a certain amount of tissue tension which resists deformation. It is not uncommon for interface pressures of around 30–40 mmHg to be seen as 'safe'. This is not always correct. Ageing causes a reduction in the numbers of elastic fibres in the tissues, resulting in reduced tissue tension. In situations where the blood pressure is artificially lowered, such as during some types of surgery, capillary pressure is also likely to be lower. In these circumstances, very little pressure is required to cause capillary occlusion. Ek *et al.* (1987) found that a pressure of only 11 mmHg was necessary to cause capillary occlusion in some hemiplegic patients.

If unrelieved pressure persists for a long period of time, tissue necrosis will follow. Prolonged pressure causes distortion of the soft-tissues and results in destruction of tissue close to the bone. A cone-shaped sore is created, with the widest part of the cone close to the bone and the narrowest on the body surface. Thus, the visible sore fails to reveal the true extent of tissue damage.

The bony prominences which are most vulnerable to pressure sore development are sometimes referred to as the pressure areas. These include: the sacrum, ischial tuberosities, trochanters, heels and elbows (see Fig.5.1).

Shear forces can deform and disrupt tissue and so damage the blood vessels. Shearing may occur if the patient slides down the bed. The skeleton and tissues nearest to it move, but the skin on the buttocks remains still. One of the main culprits of shearing is the back-rest of the bed which encourages sliding; chairs which fail to maintain a good posture may also cause shearing.

Friction occurs when two surfaces rub together. The commonest cause is when the patient is dragged rather than lifted across the bed. It causes the top layers of epithelial cells to be scraped off. Moisture exacerbates the effect of friction.

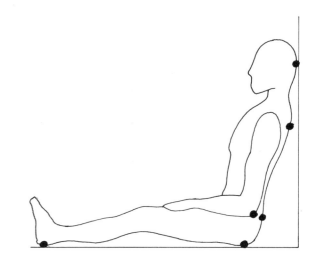

Fig. 5.1 The bony prominences or pressure areas.

Moisture may be found on a patient's skin as a result of excessive sweating or urinary incontinence.

Internal factors

The human body is frequently subjected to some or all of the external factors, but does not automatically develop pressure sores. The determining factor(s) come from within the patient.

General health is important as the body can withstand greater external pressure in health than when sick. Bliss (1990) suggests that the acutely ill are particularly vulnerable. Although the reasons for this are not certain, Bliss suggests some precipitating factors including pain, low blood pressure, heart failure, the use of sedatives, vasomotor failure, peripheral vasoconstriction due to shock, and others.

Age has been shown to be a major factor in the development of pressure sores. David *et al.* (1983) carried out a pressure sore prevalence survey of 20 health districts from within four health regions. They found that 85% of the patients with pressure sores were over 65 years old. A survey by Nyquist & Hawthorn (1987) found that within one health authority 47% of patients with pressure sores were on wards for the elderly.

As people age, their skin becomes thinner and less elastic. In part this is because the collagen in the dermis reduces in quantity and quality. Collagen provides a buffer which helps to prevent disruption of the microcirculation (Krouskop, 1983). There may be wasting of the overall body mass, resulting in loose folds of skin. There is also an increased likelihood of chronic illness or disease developing – many of which may also predispose to pressure sore development. Once a sore occurs it is much harder to heal in an older person than in a younger one (see Chapter 3).

Reduced mobility can affect the ability to relieve pressure effectively, if at all. It also predisposes to shearing and friction if the patient is confined to a bed or chair. General prevalence surveys such as those of David *et al.* (1983) and Nyquist &

Hawthorn (1987), have found reduced mobility to be a contributory factor for many patients with pressure sores. Versluysen (1986) studied 100 patients over the age of 60 years with a fractured femur and found a pressure sore prevalence of 66%. This study was replicated by Nyquist & Hawthorn (1988) who found a pressure sore prevalence of 42.3%.

Exton-Smith & Sherwin (1961) studied the number of movements made by 50 elderly patients during the night. A strong relationship was found between those with reduced movement and the development of pressure sores. Reduced movement during sleep may be associated with a variety of drugs such as hypnotics, anxiolytics, antidepressants, opioid analgesics, and antihistamines.

Another aspect of reduced mobility is that of the patient undergoing major surgery. Such operations may last many hours during which the patient lies immobile on the hard operating table. Mobility may then be reduced in the immediate postoperative period because of the effects of the anaesthetic, pain, analgesia, infusions or drains. Very sophisticated surgery is carried out these days, and often on the older patient, too. The risk of pressure sore development is consequently increased.

Reduced mobility may also be associated with neurological deficit such as a patient with paraplegia, but this is not always so: the diabetic may suffer from neuropathy without loss of mobility. Neurological deficit may be associated with strokes, multiple sclerosis, diabetes, and spinal cord injury or degeneration. Loss of sensation means the patient is unaware of the need to relieve pressure, even if he is able to do so. Dealey (1991a) found that neurological deficit was a common factor in those patients with pressure sores found in a survey of a teaching hospital.

Reduced nutritional status impairs the elasticity of the skin. Long-term it will lead to anaemia and a reduction of oxygen to the tissues. Pinchcofsky-Devin & Kaminski (1986) assessed the nutritional status of 232 patients in a nursing home. Some 117 patients had mild-to-moderate malnutrition and 17 had severe malnutrition. Although none of the other patients were affected, pressure sores were present in all the 17 severely malnourished patients. Cullum & Clark (1992) carried out a study of intrinsic factors associated with pressure sores in elderly people, and found that serum protein concentrations were significantly lower in those patients admitted with pressure sores and those who developed sores when compared with patients who did not have pressure sores. The factors which may lead to malnutrition are discussed in Chapter 3.

Body weight should also be considered. Very emaciated patients have no fatty 'padding' over bony prominences, and so have less protection against pressure. On the other hand, very obese patients are difficult to move, and unless great care is taken, they may be dragged rather than lifted in the bed, thus precipitating tissue damage. Another problem of the obese patient is that moisture from sweating may become trapped between the rolls of fat causing maceration of the skin. Both of these types of patient may also have a poor nutritional status.

Incontinence of urine can contribute to maceration of the skin and thus increase the risk of friction. Constant washing removes natural body oils, drying the skin. In a pressure sore prevalence survey of Greater Glasgow, Jordan & Clark (1977) found 15.5% of patients with pressure sores to be incontinent of urine and 39.7% to have faecal incontinence. Factors which may be associated with urinary incontinence include the use of diuretics or sedatives. Diarrhoea may cause incontinence in the elderly or immobile patient. It is a side-effect found with the use of some antibiotics. *Poor blood supply* to the periphery lowers the local capillary pressure and causes malnutrition in the tissues. It may be caused by disease, such as heart disease, peripheral vascular disease or diabetes; or drugs, such as beta-blockers and ina-tropic sympathomimetics, may cause peripheral vasoconstriction. These drugs may be used following cardiac surgery when the patient is already suffering from reduced mobility.

5.2.2 The cost of pressure sores

The true cost of pressure sores is impossible to calculate. There is the untold cost in terms of pain and suffering to the patient as well as the cost to the health service. There is little official data in the UK. Robertson *et al.* (1990) suggest that the cost of treating pressure sores could be as much as £750 million per annum. This is more than the reported cost of treating heart disease in the UK (£500 million per annum) (Durham & Grice, 1991). Waterlow (1988) suggested that the cost was rather lower, in the region of £300 million each year.

Preston (1991) calculated the cost of pressure sores in community patients in one health authority. He suggests that £250 000 is 'lost' to the health authority each year in treating these patients. Hibbs (1988) showed the cost of treating one patient with a deep sacral pressure sore was £25 905.58. This patient was in hospital for 180 days. A further calculation looked at the 'opportunity costs'. Opportunity costs describe what has been foregone because of specific circumstances. For example, because of the extended stay in hospital of this patient, the opportunity to carry out some 16 routine hip or knee replacements was lost. Similar calculations can also be made looking at standard days and standard costs. Dealey (1993) noted the cost of treating one standard pressure sore patient to be just over £22 000. The cost of a suitable mattress to prevent further tissue breakdown after discharge was £450 – indicating that prevention is cheaper than cure!

In future, with resource management, it is to be hoped that more data will be collected on the cost of pressure sores, if only to support the case for improved prevention.

5.2.3 Prevention of pressure sores

Although it is a truism, as far as pressure sores are concerned, prevention is better than cure. Waterlow (1988) suggests that 95% of all pressure sores could be prevented. The document *Health of the Nation* (Department of Health, 1992) calls for an annnual reduction of 5–10% in the incidence of pressure sores. In 1986, the Royal College of Physicians presented a report entitled 'Disability in 1986 and Beyond'. It recommended that every health district should have a pressure sore prevention and treatment service. Several outline criteria were suggested which will be discussed in turn.

1. A written policy for the prevention and management of pressure sores.
A district policy confers a recognition of the importance of pressure sore prevention which has previously been lacking. Many health authorities are establishing policies, often written in the form of standards of care – for example, the City and Hackney Health Authority (Hibbs, 1988). Although such policies should be prepared by a multidisciplinary team, nurses can play an important role. Livesley & Simpson (1993) have produced a useful guide for establishing a prevention policy in both hospital and community. The Department of Health has commissioned the Clinical Standards Advisory Group to produce guidelines for the prevention and management of pressure sores (Young, 1993).

2. The service should have a designated member of the medical staff.
In an editorial in the *Lancet*, Bliss (1990) deplored the fact that many doctors failed to take responsibility for pressure sores, seeing them instead to be a failure of nursing care. Bliss called for a greater interest by all doctors. A survey of pressure sore awareness by Kulkarni & Philbin (1993) found that only 29% of medical staff responded to the questions. This was less than among other disciplines – which the authors felt was indicative of a lack of interest in the topic. However, in many areas *geriatricians* have become involved in pressure sore prevention and management. Physicians and surgeons caring for people with spinal cord injury have also developed considerable skill and knowledge in this field.

3. A senior nurse should be responsible for running the District Pressure Sore Service. She/he should be trained in all aspects of pressure sore prevention and management and should be available for advice and training of hospital and community staff.
In some health authorities this role is combined with other duties. Livesley & Simpson (1989) suggest that it is advantageous to have a clinical nurse specialist in pressure sore management whose aims would be to define, develop, implement and evaluate a prevention policy. Gradually the value of a clinical nurse specialist is becoming recognized. As yet there is no recognized course or training for such a post. Also, the titles vary from 'Pressure Sore Advisor' to 'Clinical Nurse Specialist in Tissue Viability'. Dealey (1989b) has described one interpretation of the role: the clinical nurse specialist role provides an opportunity for nurses to develop a unique speciality which covers many areas of patient care.

4. Hospital and community nurses should have training in the prevention and management of pressure sores.
It is sad that the Royal College of Physicians' report restricts such training to nurses. It perpetuates the myth that pressure sores are a nursing domain and solely a nursing responsibility. Although it is true that nurses need the widest range of knowledge because they have the greatest patient contact, *all* health care disciplines need educating in those aspects of patient care which impinge on pressure sore development and treatment. Patients, too, require education about their responsibilities – particularly if they are likely to be at risk long-term. The United States Department of Health and Human Services (1992) have produced a reference guide for clinicians with an algorithm (Fig. 5.2) for easy reference. This is

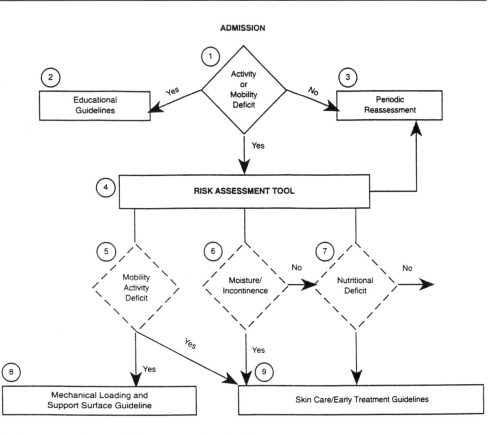

Fig. 5.2 Pressure ulcer prediction and prevention algorithm.

(From: Panel on the Prediction and Prevention of Pressure Wounds (1992), AHCPR Publication 92–0050.)

intended to educate all disciplines. A guide for patients has also been produced in order to encourage patients to be active in their own care.

> *5. Regular surveys of pressure sore prevalence and incidence in hospital and community should be undertaken.*

Before establishing any sort of prevention policy, an assessment of the size of the pressure sore problem should be made as it will provide baseline information. Further studies will then be able to acertain the effectiveness of the prevention policy. The numbers of patients with pressure sores have been measured in a number of areas and countries. The methodologies for collecting these data vary, so direct comparison cannot be made. Most of the prevalence surveys, for example, were point prevalence studies, that is a 'snap shot' carried out on a single day. Some were carried out in one hospital, others across a health authority but excluding areas such as maternity, paediatrics and acute psychiatry.

Generally speaking, the prevalence of pressure sores ranges from 4% to 14% (Ek & Boman, 1982; Warner & Hall, 1986). However, a recent report by O'Dea (1993) suggests that the figures may be higher. In a series of surveys in seven hospitals involving over 3000 patients the overall prevalence was found to be 18.6% with a range of 14.4% to 22.8%. O'Dea discusses the problems associated with the identification of grade 1 pressure sores. If they are eliminated, the prevalence is 10.1%. Table 5.1 shows some of the surveys that have been carried out and the types of patients that have been surveyed. Apart from Clark *et al.* (1978) none of these surveys measured the prevalence of pressure sores in the community. Dealey (1991a) found that 24.1% of patients with pressure sores had been admitted from the community with the sores. There is certainly a need to measure the problem in the community as well as in hospital because of the considerable drain on resources.

Although prevalence surveys provide useful baseline information, it is likely that pressure sore *incidence* will be measured in future. Incidence measures the numbers of pressure sores developing in a specific clinical area over a period of time. The Audit Commission (1991) has denoted that pressure sore incidence is one of the markers of quality of care within hospitals. The report recommends that recording the incidence of pressure sores should play an integral part in monitoring quality outcomes. Klazinga & Geibing (1993) reporting on a European quality assurance project found that measuring pressure sore incidence in a hospital over a period of time was a useful exercise.

6. Patients should be assessed using a pressure sore risk calculator to identify those at risk of developing sores.

Table 5.1 Examples of pressure sore prevalence surveys.

Researcher(s)	Date	Area	Methodology	Prevalence
Clark, Barbanel, Jordan & Nicol	1978	Greater Glasgow H.A. (excl. maternity, psychiatry, mentally handicapped).	Questionnaire; point prevalence.	8.8%
Ek & Boman	1982	Public health services area in Sweden.	Interview over one-week period.	4%
David, Chapman, Chapman & Lockett	1983	20 health districts in 4 health regions (excl. paediatrics, maternity, mental subnormality, acute psychiatry).	Structured interviews.	6.7%
Warner & Hall	1986	Hospital (excl. paediatrics).	Data collection over 4 weeks.	14%
Nyquist & Hawthorn	1987	Nottingham H.A. (excl. community, maternity, acute psychiatry).	Questionnaire; point prevalance.	5.3%
Dealey	1991	Queen Elizabeth Hospital, Birmingham	Questionnaire; point prevalence.	7.3%

In order to be able to identify patients at risk of developing pressure sores, it is helpful to use a risk calculator. This provides a means of assessing patients objectively. It should be noted that regular assessments should be made to identify changes in condition which may alter the degree of risk.

There are a number of risk calculators available. The earliest that was developed was the Norton Score (Norton *et al.*, 1975) (See Fig. 5.3). Norton studied geriatric patients and identified various factors (such as mobility) which could indicate risk of pressure sore development. Each factor was then divided into different levels and given scores. When the patient was assessed, an appropriate level for each factor was identified and a score given. The total of the five scores indicated the degree of risk of the patient: the highest score being 20 and the lowest, 5; a score of 12 or less indicated the patient is 'at risk'.

Chapman & Chapman (1986) suggested that the Norton Score was not suitable for use in younger patients. Other calculators have since been developed which attempt to refine the Norton Score (Baynes, 1984; Waterlow, 1985; Pritchard, 1986; Lowthian, 1987a). Probably the most widely used within UK hospitals is the Waterlow score (see Fig. 5.4). This calculator considers a wider range of variables than Norton. The scoring is also reversed so that the higher the score, the higher the risk. The Waterlow Score has the advantage of dividing the degree of risk into three categories: 'at risk', 'high risk' and 'very high risk'. These can be useful when considering the use of appropriate support systems. Waterlow included suggestions for preventive measures on the reverse of the card. The Braden score (Bergstrom *et al.*, 1985) is widely used in the USA. It has been demonstrated to have greater sensitivity and specificity than other scales, but only if used by registered nurses (Bergstrom *et al.*, 1987).

All of the afore-mentioned risk calculators are hospital orientated and do not readily fit into the community setting. Milward (1993) describes the Walsall pressure risk calculator which was specifically developed for community use. Like Waterlow,

PRESSURE SORE RISK CALCULATOR

SCORING SYSTEM KEY: TOTAL SCORE OF 14 AND BELOW— 'AT RISK'				
A Physical condition	**B** Mental condition	**C** Activity	**D** Mobility	**E** Incontinent
Good 4	Alert 4	Ambulant 4	Full 4	Not 4
Fair 3	Apathetic 3	Walk/Help 3	Slightly limited 3	Occasionally 3
Poor 2	Confused 2	Chairbound 2	Very limited 2	Usually/Urine 2
Very bad 1	Stuporous 1	Bedfast 1	Immobile 1	Doubly 1

Fig. 5.3 The Norton Score.

(From: Norton, D., Exton-Smith, A.N. & McLaren, R. (1975).)

WATERLOW RISK ASSESSMENT CARD

RING SCORES IN TABLE. ADD TOTAL
SEVERAL SCORES PER CATEGORY CAN BE USED

BUILD/WEIGHT FOR HEIGHT	★	RISK AREAS VISUAL SKIN TYPE	★	SEX AGE	★	SPECIAL RISKS	★
AVERAGE	0	HEALTHY	0	MALE	1	**TISSUE MALNUTRITION:**	★
ABOVE AVERAGE	1	TISSUE PAPER	1	FEMALE	2	eg. TERMINAL CACHEXIA	8
OBESE	2	DRY	1	14–49	1	CARDIAC FAILURE	5
BELOW AVERAGE	3	OEDEMATOUS	1	50–64	2	PERIPHERAL VASCULAR DISEASE	5
CONTINENCE	★	CLAMMY T↑	1	65–74	3	ANAEMIA	2
COMPLETE/ CATHETERISED	0	DISCOLOURED	2	75–80	4	SMOKING	1
						NEUROLOGICAL DEFICIT:	★
OCCASION INCONT.	1	BROKEN/SPOT	3	81 +	5	eg DIABETES, CVA	
CATH/INCONTINENT OF FAECES	2	**MOBILITY**	★	**APPETITE**	★	M.S., PARAPLEGIA;	4-6
		FULLY	0	AVERAGE	0	MOTOR/SENSORY	
DOUBLY INCONT.	3	RESTLESS/FIDGETY	1	POOR	1	**MAJOR SURGERY/TRAUMA**	★
		APATHETIC	2	N.G. TUBE/		ORTHOPAEDIC – BELOW WAIST, SPINAL	5
		RESTRICTED	3	FLUIDS ONLY	2	ON TABLE > 2 HRS	5
		INERT/TRACTION	4	NBM/ANOREXIC	3	**MEDICATION** ·	★
		CHAIRBOUND	5			STEROIDS, CYTOTOXICS, ANTI-INFLAMMATORY	4

SCORE:	10+ AT RISK	15+ HIGH RISK	20+ VERY HIGH RISK

© J WATERLOW

Fig. 5.4 The Waterlow Score.
Reproduced with permission.

the Walsall calculator includes an equipment guide to minimize inappropriate use of pressure relieving equipment.

Several criticisms have been made of *all* the risk calculators; and include the identification of patients at risk who do not subsequently develop pressure sores and failure to identify some that do develop pressure sores. For example, Goldstone & Goldstone (1982) assessed elderly orthopaedic patients using Norton. Some 89% of patients who developed pressure sores were seen to be at risk. The other 11% with pressure sores were not so identified. It can also be seen that 64% of the patients seen to be at risk did not develop pressure sores. However, the effect of nursing care may be responsible, rather than failure of the calculator. There is no way that any calculator can be truly validated without removing the influence of all nursing care, which is totally unethical. There have been no studies on the reliability of the calculators – i.e. to identify whether different nurses would achieve the same score for a patient.

Despite the criticisms that can be made of the risk calculators, there is benefit in using a systematic method of assessing and identifying patients at risk of pressure sore development. Flanagan (1993) stresses the importance of regular assessment of patients rather than just occasional assessments as part of the initial assessment of a patient. It should also be noted that once a patient is identified as being at risk, appropriate preventive action must follow. Failure to do so would put a nurse in breach of the Code of Conduct (UKCC, 1992).

7. Plastic surgeons should be available if needed.
The healing time of a large cavity pressure sore can be considerably reduced by plastic surgery. However, this is not appropriate for all patients: their condition may

be too poor or the sore may be healing rapidly. Traditionally, reconstructive plastic surgery is most commonly used on patients with spinal cord injury. Khoo & Bailey (1990) have described the principles of reconstructive surgery. They see it to be a series of steps – removal of all necrotic tissue, repeated debridement until healthy granulation tissue is obtained, and then closure of the wound using a skin graft or flap.

8. There should be a readily available supply of support systems.
Relief of pressure is the main method used in the prevention of pressure sores. This may be achieved by regular re-positioning of the patient and the use of pressure relieving equipment (support systems) when necessary. Each patient should be given care appropriate to his/her needs.

The use of positioning

For the majority of patients regular re-positioning is all that is necessary for pressure sore prevention. Patients should be moved every 2–4 hours according to need. The standard method is to turn patients from side to side. Lowthian (1979) designed a 'turning clock' to establish effective positioning. Fig. 5.5 shows how this can be used

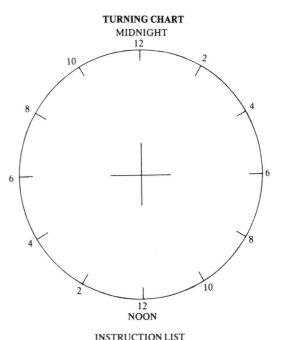

TURNING CHART
MIDNIGHT
12

12
NOON

INSTRUCTION LIST

MN - 1		7 - 8		2 - 3		9 - 10	
1 - 2		8 - 9		3 - 4		10 - 11	
2 - 3		9 - 10		4 - 5		11 - MN	
3 - 4		10 - 11		5 - 6			
4 - 5		11 - MD		6 - 7			
5 - 6		12 - 1		7 - 8			
6 - 7		1 - 2		8 - 9			

Fig. 5.5 Lowthian Turning Clock.

(From: Lowthian, P. (1979).)

effectively so that a patient can be sitting up at mealtimes and side-lying at other times. Regular assessment of the pressure areas must be made; this is in order to detect any evidence of excessive pressure. If this occurs other means of pressure relief may be needed.

However, regular turning of patients can put nurses at risk of back injury – particularly so on medical, neurological, geriatric and orthopaedic wards. One study showed that two nurses on a geriatric ward lifted the equivalent of 2.5 tons in weight in one hour (General, Municipal and Boilermakers Union, 1985)! When moving very heavy patients, hoists should be used to reduce the risk of back injury. In fact, lifting regulations have been established by a European Community directive indicating the necessity for a policy on manual lifting. In the UK the Health and Safety Executive produced such a document in 1992. It includes details of the duties of both employers and employees as well as advice procedures (Health and Safety Executive, 1992).

An alternative to traditional 'turning' of patients is the 30° tilt. This method of positioning patients was developed in a younger disabled unit (Preston, 1988). The patient is placed into a tilted position by the use of pillows (see Fig. 5.6). Once in position, there is no pressure on the sacrum or heels. The interface pressure on the

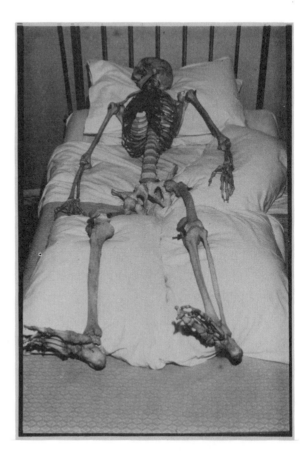

Fig. 5.6 The 30° tilt demonstrated by an anatomical skeleton.

buttock is around 25 mmHg. The patient can be left for increasingly longer periods without turning, again careful observation must be made of all vulnerable areas. Once a patient has become accustomed to using the 30° tilt, she/he may be left for up to eight hours without turning. Not only does this allow a patient to have an undisturbed night's sleep, but it is also of great benefit for use in the community. This method of positioning is not suitable for all patients, however, although it is a useful addition to the skills available for preventing pressure sores.

The standard hospital mattress

Much has been written in recent years about the use of various support systems; far less time has been spent considering the standard mattress – despite the fact that this is what most patients use. O'Dea (1993) found that 33% of patients with pressure damage were being nursed on a standard hospital mattress, which is made of foam. Foam has a finite life-span: the Department of Health recommends that the standard mattress should have a life-span of four years. All hospitals should establish a replacement programme. Mattresses need to be tested annually for grounding and the effectiveness of the cover. Worn out mattresses can then be replaced.

The foam in the mattresses should be at least 130 mm thick, or they will collapse in a much shorter time. The use of two-way stretch covers gives improved pressure relief, and this is in contrast to the Staph Chek covers which increase pressure (Podmore, 1993). Damage to the mattress and water resistance of the cover can be minimized by avoiding the use of alcohol sprays in cleaning and using soap and water instead.

Pressure-relieving beds and mattresses

There is an ever-increasing range of equipment available for use in relieving pressure. These range from mattress overlays to highly sophisticated beds. They have a variety of characteristics and include air-filled or water-filled mattresses, floatation gels, hollow core fibres or foams. Some reduce pressure by distributing the patients weight more evenly and reducing pressures over bony prominences; others actually relieve pressure, in a variety of ways.

However, caution is needed in the purchase of pressure-relieving equipment. Clark & Cullum (1992) found that, despite an increase in the availability of equipment, the prevalence of pressure sores actually increased over a four-year period. Young (1992) and Bliss & Thomas (1993a) have discussed the lack of research into the various pressure-relieving systems available. Bliss & Thomas (1993b, 1993c) provide an overview of such clinical trials that have been conducted.

Until more conclusive evidence is produced, selection of a support system must depend upon the degree of risk of pressure sores to the patient, and individual choice. Dealey (1990) has reviewed the range of support systems and identified their potential use. In many areas, choice is limited according to the availability of equipment. Table 5.2 suggests how equipment can be selected according to the degree of risk of the patient. Appendix B gives further information about the different types of support systems.

Table 5.2 Selecting a support system according to the degree of risk of the patient.

Low-risk patients	
	Hollow core fibre overlays
	Bead overlays
	Gel pads
	Foam overlays
Medium-risk patients	
	Foam overlays
	Foam replacement mattresses
	Static air mattress
	Combination foam/water mattresses
	Combination foam/gel mattresses
	Water beds
	Alternating air pads
	Double-layer alternating air mattress
High-risk patients	
	Double-layer alternating air mattress
	Air floatation pads
	Dynamic air floatation mattress
	Air wave mattress
	Low air loss bed
	Air fluidized bed

Turning beds are particularly useful for very heavy patients or for patients in the community who cannot be turned at night-time. There are various systems that can be used. One type is a bed made of long sections which lift alternately on either side to tilt the patient. Electronic controls allow the programme to be preset and the patient to be moved every 2–4 hours according to need. Other systems are based on inflatable bolsters lying under the mattress along the length of the bed. Again, they are controlled electronically to inflate and deflate alternately.

Additions to the bed

Pressure relief can be enhanced by the use of simple measures. The use of bed cradles can lift the weight of the bed clothes off the patient, thus relieving over-all weight on the mattress, and also allowing the patient to move a little on his/her own accord, if possible. Back-rests are widely used, but it should be remembered that they cause the patient to slide down the bed, thus risking damage to the skin by shearing. Strategic placing of pillows can relieve pressure from bony prominences such as heels, the malleoli of the ankles, and the knees. Pads can be applied to the heels or elbows for extra pressure relief. If the patient is out of bed during the day, these pads can be applied at night. Sheepskins are very widely used. They do not provide pressure relief, but reduce the risk of friction and absorb moisture. Constant washing makes them rather matted and this may actually cause pressure problems. They need to be regularly replaced or other types of pressure relief should be used.

Chairs

Once an ill patient starts to be sat out of bed, she/he is perceived to be 'mobile' and so may be left in the chair for long periods of time without actually being moved. Many hospital armchairs are in a poor state and fail to give any pressure relief or to maintain a good posture (Dealey et al., 1991). Chairs should be checked and replaced or repaired in the same way as mattresses. Many chairs have a reclining back of between 15° and 40° which puts the patient in a semireclining posture. This may make it more difficult for the patient to get up. Ideally, a chair should have a recline of not more than 10° enabling the patient to move more freely. Although cushions may be added to chairs to improve pressure relief, the cushion should not make the chair so high that the patient's feet do not touch the floor. Conventional seating is not suitable for everyone. Some patients have severe seating problems due to contractures, deformity or infirmity. Specialized seating must be considered for these people.

Cushions

Most of the research on cushions has been on those for use in wheelchairs. Wheelchairs have a canvas base which Rithalia (1989) found exerted pressures in the region of 226 mmHg. It is essential, therefore, that a cushion should *always* be used in a wheelchair. For those who become wheelchair-bound because of disability, special assessment should be made to identify the cushion most suited to the specific needs of that person. Many physiotherapists and occupational therapists have developed specialist skills in such an assessment. There are a wide range of cushions available, and they are made from materials similar to those used for mattresses and overlays.

Other hospital equipment

Vulnerable patients may spend time lying or sitting on very hard surfaces such as operating tables, X-ray tables, trolleys and some types of wheelchair. Very little consideration has been given to the need to provide some sort of pressure relief in these circumstances. Versluysen (1986) undertook a study of 100 consecutive elderly patients admitted with a fractured femur. The interface pressures were measured on the casualty trolleys and operating tables. The casualty trolleys with a 5 cm deep foam mattress showed pressures ranging from 56–50 mmHg at the sacrum to 150–160 mmHg at the heels. The fracture operating table had interface pressures ranging from 75–80 mmHg at the sacrum to 60–120 mmHg at the heels. Bridel (1993) conducted a small pilot study of 24 patients undergoing surgery. She found an incidence of 12.5% of pressure sores that occurred as a result of damage on the operating table. Lowthian (1989) has described some of the methods of padding used with trolleys and operating tables used at the Royal National Orthopaedic Hospital, Stanmore. This is an area where considerably more research is required, particularly into strategies to reduce pressure.

Summary

The various aspects of pressure sore prevention can be summarized as follows:

Assessment: identify those at risk using a risk calculator.
Consider the nutritional status of patient(s).
Identify continence problems.
Monitor all support systems, establishing replacement or main-tenance programmes where appropriate.

Planning: Instigate a personal pressure-sore prevention programme for all at-risk patients, including appropriate methods of pressure relief and management of specific problems.
Ensure staff have an adequate knowledge of causes and prevention of pressure sores.
Establish a teaching programme for long-term at-risk patients and their carers.

Evaluation: Reassess all patients regularly to identify changes in degree of risk.
Check vulnerable skin areas of all at-risk patients regularly. This may be undertaken by nurse, patient or carer.
Conduct regular surveys of prevalence and incidence of pressure sores.
Monitoring of usage of support systems.

5.2.4 Management of pressure sores

If a pressure sore occurs, preventive measures should still be continued. The precise cause of the sore and the effectiveness of the prevention programme need to be evaluated. Any necessary changes must be made, such as using a different support system or increasing proteins and vitamins in the patient's diet. There are several other factors which also need to be considered in the management of pressure sores. These include the position of the sore, grading of the sore and its appearance, and appropriate selection of wound management products.

The position of pressure sores

Some bony prominences are more prone to pressure sores than others. Lockett (1983) reported on the position of pressure sores found in the survey by David *et al.* (1983). Fig. 5.7 shows the range of positions with the percentages found in each. The findings indicate that there are some specific aspects of care that need to be considered.

Sacrum: Dressings must be chosen with care, as many tend to ruckle up as the patient moves. Chair sitting must be strictly regulated as to type of chair and length of time seated in it.

Buttocks: As for sacrum.

Heels: Ideally, dressings must not be too bulky as this may impede mobility. Dressings may need to be 'tailored' in order to fit around the heel correctly. If

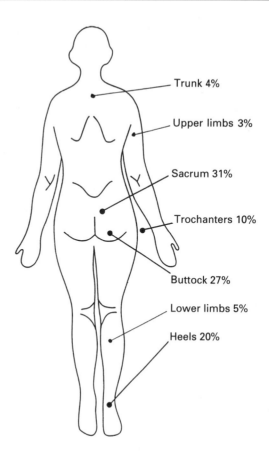

Trunk 4%

Upper limbs 3%

Sacrum 31%

Trochanters 10%

Buttock 27%

Lower limbs 5%

Heels 20%

Fig. 5.7 The common position of pressure sores.
(After Lockett, 1983.)

footware is being worn, care must be taken to ensure that it is not too tight, or this will exert pressure on the heel. Ensure there is adequate pressure relief when in bed.
Trochanters: Some dressings may ruckle up, so select carefully.
Elbows: Pressure sores are usually caused by friction from moving about the bed. Consider ways of reducing friction – e.g. use of a monkey pole, use of pads or semipermeable film dressings.
Trunk: Sores here are uncommon, so try and identify source of pressure and remove or modify it.

Grading of pressure sores

Use of a recognized system of grading pressure sores can be helpful by providing objective descriptions of sores. It also gives a more accurate picture of the amount of tissue damage. The grading system should be used in conjunction with other descriptive tools, such as measuring or tracing the sore, and describing its appearance.

Several methods of grading pressure sores have been put forward. Some incorporate four grades (Clark *et al.*, 1978; David *et al.*, 1983; McClement, 1984).

Each method varies slightly, but in all cases the higher the grade, the deeper the sore. Torrance (1983) suggested a five-grade system and Lowthian (1987b) suggested six grades. Ideally there should be one recognized grading system. The American National Pressure Ulcer Advisory Panel (1989) produced a Consensus Development Statement which proposed a grading system that was an amalgamation of several commonly used methods of grading. They proposed it should be the start of developing a universally accepted grading system.It is as follows:

Stage I: Non-blanchable erythema of intact skin, heralding skin ulceration.
Stage II: Partial-thickness skin loss involving epidermis and/or dermis. The ulcer is superficial and may be seen as a blister, abrasion or crater.
Stage III: Full-thickness wound involving epidermis, dermis and subcuticular layer. The ulcer presents as a crater with or without undermining.
Stage IV: Extensive destruction involving other tissues such as muscle, tendon or bone.

Plates 10, 11, 12 and 13 show examples of each of these grades of pressure sore.

Pressure sore appearance

Wound appearance has been discussed in detail in Chapter 4. The same principles can be applied to pressure sores. A pressure sore should be assessed for its appearance as well as its grade. For example, Stages III and IV sores can be necrotic, infected, sloughy or granulating in appearance. Accurate assessment is necessary in order to select a suitable wound management product.

Selection of wound management products

A variety of wound management products can be used when treating pressure sores. The range of wound management products available is discussed in Section 2.6. The appropriate use of these products is discussed in further detail in Section 4.2. As standards of care and policies are being developed in relation to pressure sore management it is helpful to have some guidelines for dressing selection. Fig. 5.8 gives suggestions in broad terms which can be adapted according to the needs of the individual areas.

5.3 THE MANAGEMENT OF LEG ULCERS

Leg ulcers are an increasingly common chronic wound and have been recognized for many years. Those following the Hippocratic view that disease was the result of imbalance of the four humours of the body, believed that a leg ulcer allowed the bad humours to leach out. In some areas, this belief still persists – the ulcer lets the bad out and if it heals the person will die. In such circumstances there may be little incentive to conform to treatment.

Until recently there was little interest among doctors in the treatment of this

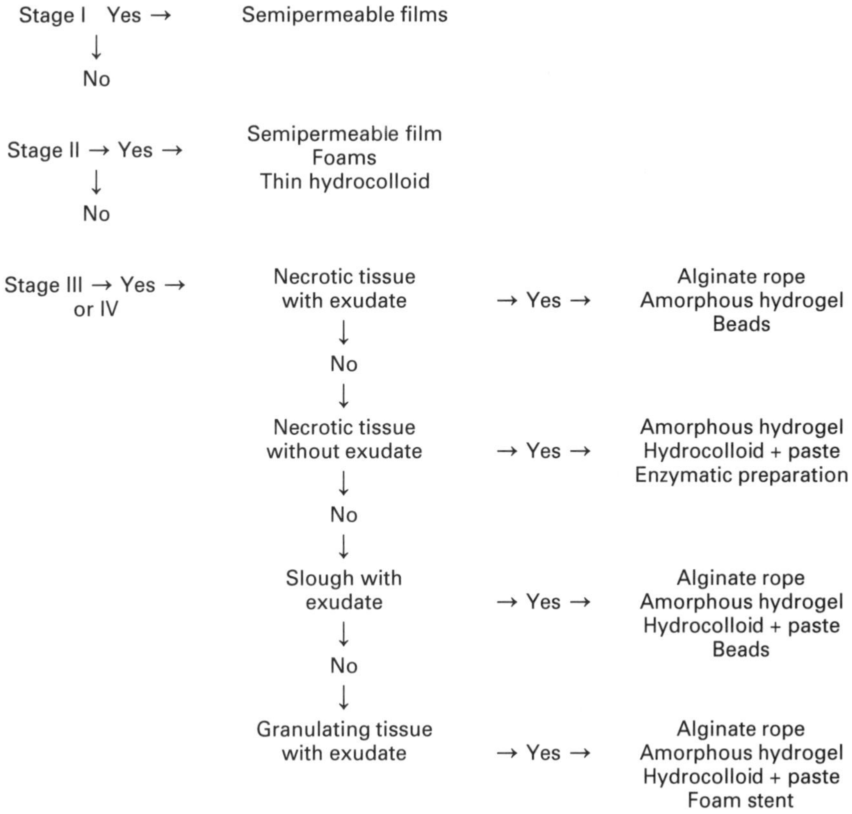

Stage I Yes → Semipermeable films
↓
No

Stage II → Yes → Semipermeable film
↓ Foams
No Thin hydrocolloid

Stage III → Yes → Necrotic tissue → Yes → Alginate rope
or IV with exudate Amorphous hydrogel
↓ Beads
No
↓
Necrotic tissue → Yes → Amorphous hydrogel
without exudate Hydrocolloid + paste
↓ Enzymatic preparation
No
↓
Slough with → Yes → Alginate rope
exudate Amorphous hydrogel
↓ Hydrocolloid + paste
No Beads
↓
Granulating tissue → Yes → Alginate rope
with exudate Amorphous hydrogel
Hydrocolloid + paste
Foam stent

Fig. 5.8 Choosing appropriate wound management products for pressure sores.

condition; their views seemed to coincide with that of an eighteenth-century physician who described the care of leg ulcers as 'an unpleasant and inglorious task where much labour must be bestowed and little honour gained' (quoted in Loudon, 1982). Modern developments in wound management have revitalized those caring for patients with leg ulcers.

5.3.1 The epidemiology of leg ulcers

There have been two major surveys carried out in the UK to ascertain the number of people with leg ulcers. The largest was the Lothian and Forth Valley survey in Scotland (Callam et al., 1985). They found eight people with leg ulcers per thousand of the population: 10 per thousand of the adult population and 36 per thousand of the population over the age of 65 years. They also found that the prevalence increased with age. Cornwall et al. (1986) surveyed an urban London health district and found 38 per ten thousand people with leg ulcers. Dale & Gibson (1986) extrapolated the figures from the Scottish survey and calculated that in the UK there are 440 000 people who could potentially develop ulcers and about

88 000 people with open ulcers. Gilchrist (1989) suggests that the number of people receiving treatment for leg ulcers is about 400 000.

Leg ulcers are predominantly seen to be a condition affecting women. Up to the age of 40, ulcers are fairly equally distributed between the sexes. At the age range of 65–74 years, the female/male ratio is 2.6:1. This increases to a ratio of 10.3:1 over the age of 85 (Dale & Gibson, 1986). This difference is probably, in part, because women live longer than men. It may also be because of the increased risk of deep vein thrombosis during pregnancy.

One of the problematic features of leg ulcers is the length of time they can take to heal and the frequency of recurrence. Dale & Gibson (1986) describe the findings in the Lothian and Forth Valley survey. They note that 21% of ulcers were healed in up to 3 months, 29% took 3–12 months, 40% took 1–5 years and 10% took over 5 years to heal. One unfortunate person had had an open ulcer for 62 years. Nearly half the patients had between 2 and 5 episodes of ulceration and 21% had over 6 episodes of ulceration.

5.3.2 The cost of leg ulcers

As has been shown, leg ulcers can be a longstanding and recurrent problem. Inevitably, they are also very expensive to manage. The majority are cared for in the community and so require home visits or special trips to clinics. Harkiss (1985) was one of the first to undertake comparative costs of different types of treatment. Although the figures are now dated, it is interesting to note that many of the modern dressings are cheaper to use than more traditional treatments. Thomas (1990a) takes a more global view and suggests the overall costs to the health service are in the region of £300–£600 million each year. Bosanquet (1992) puts the cost at £400 million a year.

Milward (1988) approached the problem of costs from a different angle and considered the savings which could be made when effective treatment was used. The figures related to 26 patients with leg ulcers whose progress was recorded over a three-month period. Initially, all the patients were receiving a daily visit from the community nurse. Once effective treatment was implemented, the number of visits each week were reduced, by varying amounts, for all but three patients. The total number of 'saved' visits amounted to 990. The cost saving in time and materials was calculated to be £14 572.80. If these figures were projected over a year, the potential savings could be in the region of £58 000. These figures do not take into consideration the fact that some of the ulcers may have healed in this time and that other patients may be referred for treatment.

Leg ulcers can be seen as an expensive disease, but potential savings can be made when cost-effective care is instigated.

5.3.3 The causes of leg ulcers

There are a variety of causes of leg ulcers. The commonest are venous disease, arterial disease or a combination of the two – when the ulcers are generally referred to as 'mixed ulcers'. Another common cause is diabetes. The aetiology and the management of each of these types of ulcer will be considered in turn.

Other causes of leg ulceration are infection, neoplasms, inflammatory disease and trauma.

5.3.4 Venous ulceration

Aetiology

Chronic venous insufficiency is the commonest cause of leg ulcers. Callam *et al.* (1985) found that 70% of the ulcers that they surveyed were of venous origin. Initially, thrombosis or varicosity causes damage to the valves in the veins of the leg. The deep vein is surrounded by muscle. When the leg is exercised, the calf muscle contracts and squeezes the veins, encouraging the flow of blood along the vein. This is often referred to as the calf muscle pump.

Normally blood flows from the superficial veins to the deep veins via a series of perforator vessels. The valves in the vessels ensure that blood moves from the capillary bed towards the heart (see Fig. 5.9). If some of the valves become damaged then blood can flow in either direction. The backflow of blood towards the capillary bed leads to venous hypertension. As a result, the capillaries become distorted and more permeable. Larger molecules than normal are able to escape into the extravascular space, for example fibrinogen and red blood cells. The haemoglobin is first released from the red blood cells and then broken down causing eczema and and a brown staining in the gaiter area. This condition is called lipodermato-sclerosis. The slightest trauma to the leg and an ulcer will develop. Common

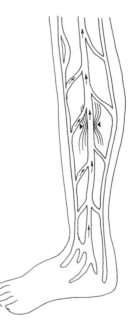

Fig. 5.9 The veins of the leg.

examples of trauma are knocking the leg on the corner of a piece of furniture or a fall, injuring the lower leg.

Burnand (1988) was the first to describe a fibrin cuff around the capillaries. He postulated that it was formed from fibrinogen leaking from the capillaries and that it blocked oxygen and nutrients reaching the tissues and the removal of waste products. Therefore, the fibrin cuff could be seen as a precursor to lipodermato- sclerosis. A small study by Eaglestein et al. (1988) supported some of this hypothesis. They found low levels of transcutaneous oxygen adjacent to the site of venous ulcers. They also found that the more severe the lipodermatosclerosis, the more difficult it was for the ulcers to be healed .

The lymphatic system may also be affected. The lymphatics are responsible for removing protein, fat, cells and excess fluid from the tissues. Ryan (1987) has described how the superficial lymphatics in the dermis disappear. This results in waste products accumulating in the tissues which can cause fibrosis and further oedema.

● *Assessment* ●

Full assessment of the patient is essential as many factors can delay the healing of chronic wounds (see Chapter 3). A medical assessment may be necessary to ensure accurate diagnosis. Factors that may need to be particularly considered include nutritional status, mobility, sleeping, blood and urine testing to screen for anaemia and diabetes, pain, the psychological effects of leg ulceration and the patient's understanding of the disease process. The past medical history may give an indi- cation of any causative factors, such as a previous deep vein thrombosis. A history of cardiovascular or rheumatoid disease may be indicative of other problems. A comprehensive assessment of the affected leg must be made, as it is important to rule out arterial disease. The treatments for these two types of ulcer are not compatable.

First look at the legs. The characteristic staining of lipodermatosclerosis is usually clearly seen in the gaiter area. Ankle flare may also be present. This is distension of the network of small veins situated just below the medial malleolus. Oedema may be present, but can also be found in arterial ulceration. Theoretically, the leg and foot should feel warm to touch, but if the weather is cold this may not be the case. The skin surrounding the ulcer may be fragile and eczematous.

Typically, venous ulcers are found on or near the medial malleolus. They tend to be shallow and develop slowly over a period of time. Although the pain the sufferer may feel is relatively mild, it will be increased if there is any infection in the ulcer. The ulcer appearance should be assessed as in Section 4.1. Many venous ulcers have a heavy exudate. Plate 14 shows a typical venous ulcer with staining in the gaiter area.

Differential diagnosis between venous and arterial ulcers can be made by assessing the blood supply to the leg. This may be done in a variety of ways. The easiest is to take the pedal pulses which can be found in the midline of the dorsum of the foot. However, if oedema is present they may be difficult to find. More and more nurses are beginning to use the doppler to assess the blood supply to the leg. It is used to compare the blood pressure in the lower leg to the brachial pressure. It is usually presented in the form of a ratio, the ankle pressure index (API), which is calculated by the following formula:

$$\frac{\text{Ankle systolic pressure}}{\text{Brachial systolic pressure}} = \text{Ankle pressure index}$$

An API of 0.9 or above indicates a normal arterial supply to the leg. If it is below 0.9 then some ischaemia is present. Compression therapy should not be used if the API is below 0.8. If there is any doubt about the presence of arterial disease, further medical opinion should be sought.

● *Planning* ●

There are two aspects to the management of venous ulcers: improving the drainage of the leg and the use of appropriate wound management products. Neither will be truly effective without the other.

The drainage of the legs can be improved in several ways: exercise, compression and elevation. The use of exercise stimulates the calf muscle pump, promoting drainage. Allen (1983) recommends that patients should walk as much as they are able and, if standing still, move from one foot to the other. He also suggests that frequent ankle exercises should be performed when sitting. Obviously exercise should be tailored to the abilities of the patient. Regular encouragement will be needed to ensure patients persist with their exercises.

Compression works with exercise to aid drainage from the superficial veins. It should be graduated so that there is a higher pressure at the ankle than at the calf. It can be achieved by the use of either bandages or stockings. Bandages are probably easiest to use in the early stages when the dressings may be rather bulky. Some remain in place day and night whereas others may be removed at night. When applying bandages it is best done before rising when the leg has the least amount of oedema.

Thomas (1990b) has categorized compression bandages into four groups:

● Light compression giving 14–17 mmHg at the ankle.
● Moderate compression giving 18–24 mmHg at the ankle.
● High compression giving 25–35 mmHg at the ankle.
● Extra high compression giving 60 mmHg at the ankle.

The level of compression needed for venous ulceration is around 40 mmHg, (Stemmer, 1969) . Therefore, the high compression bandages should be suitable. However, these pressures are dependent on the size of the limb. A large limb, swollen with oedema, would require a higher compression bandage than a thinner limb in order to achieve an adequate level of compression. There is also considerable skill in applying a compression bandage correctly and it is regrettable that bandaging is often not included in the curriculum for nurse training. Logan *et al.* (1992) found inconsistency in application among inexperienced bandagers when compared with more experienced staff. Magazinovic *et al.* (1993) found registered nurses lacked understanding of the principles of bandaging. The manufacturer's

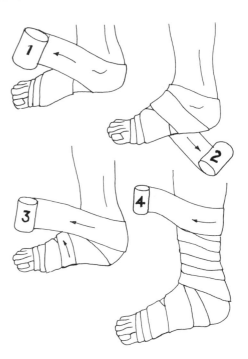

Fig. 5.10 Application of a pressure bandage.

instructions should always be followed when applying any bandage. The commonest method is to apply the bandage in a spiral, as shown in Fig. 5.10.

Blair *et al.* (1988) have used a four-layer bandage system to provide sustained compression. They found it to be an effective method of treatment. Moffatt & Dickson (1993) provide clear instruction for the use and application of this system.

Tubular bandages may also be used to provide compression. The straight variety do not give appropriate compression as it is higher at the calf than the ankle. There is a shaped tubular bandage which can be most useful as it is relatively easy to apply. This type of compression may be the easiest to pull on for someone with arthritic hands. It is more effective to use two layers of bandage.

Below-knee compression stockings are widely used as the ulcer improves and after healing. Some manufacturers also produce compression socks for men which look like ordinary socks. For many patients, socks and stockings are easier to apply than bandages. Dale & Gibson (1990) have reviewed the use of compression stockings. The British Standards Institute have specified three classes of stockings which are available on prescription. The three classes provide different ranges of compression at the ankle:

- Class I has pressures of 14–18 mmHg
- Class II has pressures of 18–24 mmHg
- Class III has pressures of 25–35 mmHg

It is very important that the patient should be correctly fitted for a stocking. Class II may be appropriate for many patients. If a Class III stocking is required, but the patient is unable or unwilling to pull them on, it may be better to use two layers of

Class I stockings. Fentem (1986) has shown that this would provide the same level of compression. Compliance is essential for this form of treatment. Mayberry *et al.* (1991) were able to achieve 97% healing with patients who were compliant and wore their compression stockings, but only 55% healing in those who were not compliant.

Patients are usually prescribed two pairs of stockings so that they have 'one to wash and one to wear'. This will get the maximum wear out of the stocking. Dale & Gibson (1990) suggest that the stockings should be washed by hand after each wearing. Thus, the stocking should have a life-span of three to four months before being replaced.

Another method of applying compression which can be used, particularly if oedema is present, is pneumatic compression. It may be applied once or twice a day for periods of up to an hour. Initially the time should be shorter and gradually increased. Although this may be a useful form of treatment, it is difficult in the community where there is limited access to such equipment. The use of pneumatic compression should be seen as an addition to the treatment regime rather than an alternative. Mulder *et al.* (1990) studied the use of sequential pneumatic compression in 10 patients with chronic venous ulcers; it was used in addition to paste bandages and compression bandages. They found that the use of pneumatic compression significantly reduced healing time.

Elevation of the legs will also help as it allows gravity to aid venous return. However, many people tend to place their feet on a low stool which is of no benefit whatsoever. To be effective, elevation of the feet should be higher than the heart. If there is an acute exacerbation of the ulcer with oedema and heavy exudate, it may be worthwhile to admit the patient to hospital so that she/he may have a short period of bedrest. Bedrest with elevation of the foot of the bed can significantly reduce oedema and improve venous return. It should not be considered as a long-term measure, however, because the ulcer will merely break down again once the patient is up and about. It may also seriously affect the mobility of older patients.

A more practical method at home is to raise the foot of the bed so that the patient's legs are elevated at night time. This may be achieved by the use of bricks or blocks of wood. The patient should also be encouraged to elevate the legs for periods during the day. Ryan (1987) describes the use of a 'Legs Up' chart (Fig. 5.11) to encourage patients to elevate their legs for at least two hours during the day. The intention is to actively involve patients in their own care.

The use of drug therapy to improve chronic venous insufficiency and healing of the ulcer has been studied. A recent study by Colgan *et al.* (1990) suggests that the use of oxypentifylline can assist in the healing of venous ulcers, but further study is required to determine it's precise action.

Management of the ulcer involves cleansing and a suitable topical application. Consideration must be given to the presence of eczema, scaling on the legs around the ulcer, wound infection, and any allergies to treatment.

Cleansing is an important factor as many patients may have been told in the past that they must never get their ulcer wet. As a result they may have not had a bath for years. Foot baths are very useful as they allow the patient to give the affected leg a good soak. Plain tap water is suitable for most patients. Attention needs to be paid

HELPING TO HEAL YOUR LEG ULCER.

If you have a venous leg ulcer, you can contribute immensely to the rate at which it heals simply by keeping your feet up every day as part of your routine.

By sitting for a short time each day in a comfortable 'legs up' position, as illustrated below, you can help your nurse to heal the wound.

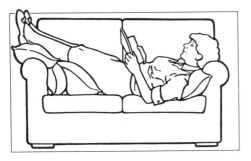

Simply record on the chart overleaf the number of hours that you have spent in the 'legs up' position each day. When the chart is full, give it back to your nurse.

The nurse will then be able to tell you if you are resting your legs enough to ensure a speedy recovery.

Fig. 5.11 'Legs up' chart.

From: Ryan T.J. (1987) *The Management of Leg Ulcers*. 2nd ed. Oxford University Press, Oxford.
By courtesy of Prof. T.J. Ryan.

PATIENT 'LEGS UP' RECORD CHART

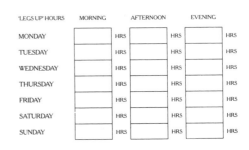

NAME   DATE

Enter in each square below the number of hours you have rested with your legs up.

'LEGS UP' HOURS	MORNING	AFTERNOON	EVENING
MONDAY	HRS	HRS	HRS
TUESDAY	HRS	HRS	HRS
WEDNESDAY	HRS	HRS	HRS
THURSDAY	HRS	HRS	HRS
FRIDAY	HRS	HRS	HRS
SATURDAY	HRS	HRS	HRS
SUNDAY	HRS	HRS	HRS

REMEMBER TO GIVE BACK THE COMPLETED CHART TO YOUR NURSE.

to the adequate cleansing of the foot bath after use. If the patient has weeping eczema, a potassium permanganate 0.01% solution can be used. It has a slightly astringent effect. It can also be applied in the form of soaks, but this is very expensive in nursing time.

Paste bandages are widely used in the treatment of leg ulcers. They are cotton bandages impregnated with different types of paste according to the manufacturer. They are soothing to sore, eczematous legs and will also lift off some of the scales that tend to form around the ulcer. Paste bandages do not provide compression, but they enhance the effect of the compression bandages used over the top. Paste bandages have to be applied in such a way as to allow for any swelling of the leg. This may be achieved by making a pleat on each turn at the front of the leg. An alternative method is to overlap each turn and cut the bandage. Paste bandages can be left in place for up to a week.

Another method of removing scales around the ulcer is the use of hydrocolloid dressings. These hydrate the skin and so lift off the scales. A slightly larger dressing than necessary can be used. Simple or bland emollients may also be used.

When taking an initial history, any reported allergies should be noted. Many long-term leg ulcer sufferers develop allergies to their treatment. Cameron (1990) patch-tested 52 patients with venous ulcers; 30 (57%) patients had an allergic reaction and of these patients, 26 had multiple reactions. Some allergens are found in creams and paste bandages such as wool alcohols, parabens and cetystearyl alcohol. Others may be found in bandages or stockings such as ester gum resin, colophony, carba mix, thiurum mix and mercapto mix. Care must be taken when using any potentially allergenic agent. It may be useful to apply a small strip of dressing to the ulcer before use as a tester, particularly when using paste bandages.

As with any wound, bacteria colonize the ulcer surface. This has been previously discussed in Section 4.2. If there is any indication of infection and/or cellulitis, medical opinion should be requested. One particular pathogenic organism which gives cause for concern in leg ulcers is β-haemolytic streptococcus. Schraibman (1987) described the relationship between the organism and giant ulcers which did not readily respond to treatment. He suggests systemic antibiotics to eliminate the bacteria and then skin grafting.

Management of the ulcer depends on the assessment and the factors previously discussed. Selection of suitable dressings is discussed in Section 4.2. Recently there have been several clinical trials of modern products on leg ulcers which have shown the effectiveness of their use. Alginates, beads, hydrocolloids and hydrogels may be particularly effective. It should be remembered that although the ulcer may be new to the nurse, the patient may have lived with it for some time. There may therefore be a credibility gap as the patient starts yet another course of treatment which, she is told, will definitely resolve the problem. Effective communication is essential to ensure that the patient understands and is prepared to comply with treatment.

• Evaluation •

Regular assessment of the ulcer may be done by the use of tracings or photographs. They are essential to monitor the progress of the ulcer. If there appears to be no progress over a period of 2–3 months the ulcer should be re-assessed and any ischaemia or infection ruled out. Patient assessment will identify any relevant factors such as loss of appetite.

If the skin on the leg tends to be scaly, a simple emollient should be used to remove the scales. Many patients complain of irritation and the action of applying emollients can help to prevent scratching.

Once the ulcer is healed, the patient should be encouraged to continue to wear compression stockings and take exercise. This is essential in preventing recurrence of ulceration. Mayberry et al. (1991) followed up 78 patients after healing of their ulcers. Some 58 (79%) were compliant and wore their compression stockings. There was an ulcer recurrence rate of 16%; in other words, 84% of ulcers remained healed. However, there was 100% recurrence within three years for those who failed to comply. Mayberry et al. suggest that these results raise questions about the possible value of surgical intervention such as ligation of perforator veins. They compare their results with published surgical studies. One example is that of Negus & Friedgood (1983) who studied 77 patients who had surgery followed by the wearing of compression stockings. They found that 84.3% remained healed, some after a three year follow-up. In the light of the Mayberry study, it is not unreasonable to ask whether Negus & Friedgood would have had the same results if their patients had not worn compression stockings.

Patients still need to be seen regularly once the ulcer is healed in order to provide encouragement and to ensure that the preventive care is understood. They should also be given information on how to get further help if the ulcer recurs. The sooner appropriate care can be given, the sooner the ulcer will heal. Prevention is obviously better than cure. If lipodermatosclerosis is observed, the person should be encouraged to wear compression stockings. Patient education is essential for full understanding of the potential hazard of ulceration. Screening programmes – where blood pressure, urine and other similar checks are made – would be an ideal opportunity to check for evidence of lipodermatosclerosis.

5.3.5 Arterial ulcers

Aetiology

Arterial ulcers are the result of inadequate tissue perfusion to the feet or legs. This is due to complete or partial blockage of the arterial supply to the legs and the underlying condition is often referred to as peripheral vascular disease. This is a general term to encompass disease which reduces the blood supply to the periphery. The commonest disease is arteriosclerosis where the artery walls become thickened. It is usually found in combination with atherosclerosis – the formation of plaques on the inner lining of the vessels. The lumen of the vessels gradually narrows causing ischaemia in the surrounding tissue, ultimately resulting in necrosis. This type of arterial insufficiency is most commonly found in men over the age of 50.

Buerger's disease is another type of disease affecting the peripheral arteries. Inflammation of the vessels results in thrombus formation and occlusion of the vessels. It is associated with heavy smoking and is found most commonly in men between the ages of twenty and thirty-five years. Ulceration associated with necrosis and gangrene may develop.

● *Assessment* ●

Assessment of the patient may reveal pain – particularly on walking – which is relieved by resting. This is known as intermittent claudication. Pain may also occur at night when the patient is in bed and can be relieved by hanging the legs down over the side of the bed. Past medical history may reveal known peripheral vascular disease or arterial surgery. A past or present history of smoking should also be noted.

On examination, the legs may feel cold to touch and have a shiny, hairless appearance. The toe nails may be thickened and opaque. The legs become white when elevated and develop a reddish/blue colour when dependent. Pedal pulses are diminished or absent. Doppler examination will reveal the presence of ischaemia with an API below 0.9. If the patient has intermittent claudication, the API is likely to be between 0.5 and 0.9. If it is below 0.5, rest pain is also likely to be present. The patient should be referred to a vascular surgeon.

The ulcer may occur anywhere on the leg or foot but most are found on the foot. The ulcer has a punched out appearance and may be deep, involving muscles or tendons. Necrosis is often present and there is far less exudate than in venous leg ulcers (see Plate 15). (Table 5.3 compares venous and arterial ulcers (Dealey, 1991b).)

● *Planning* ●

Arterial ulcers are notoriously difficult to heal and there is considerable risk of the onset of worsening gangrene and even septicaemia. Amputation of the limb may be the only solution for some. Arterial surgery to improve the blood supply may be necessary before an ulcer will heal. Early referral for reconstructive surgery is ideal. However, good management will optimize healing rates.

If a patient has severe resting pain, good pain control is an essential part of the management. The patient should also be encouraged to give up smoking as failure

Table 5.3 A comparison of venous and arterial ulcers.

Sign/symptom	Venous ulcer	Arterial ulcer
Site:	On/near medial malliolus	May be on toes, foot, heel or lateral aspect of leg.
Development:	Develops slowly	Develops rapidly
Appearance of ulcer:	Shallow margin; deep tissues not affected.	Often deep with involvement of muscle or tendons.
Appearance of leg:	Brown, varicose staining and eczema, warm to touch.	Shiny skin, cold to touch, white on elevation, may become blue when dependent.
Oedema:	Present – usually worse at end of day	Only present if patient is immobile – stasis oedema
Pain:	Pain varies, but mostly associated with oedema and infection.	Very painful. May cause waking at night, relieved by hanging leg over side of bed.
Foot pulses:	Present.	Diminished or absent.
Medical history:	DVT, phlebitis, varicose veins.	Peripheral vascular disease; ischaemic heart disease; diabetes mellitus.

From: Dealey, C. (1991b).

to do so will further compromise the blood supply to the leg. Gentle exercise will help to encourage the development of a collateral supply to the limb, thus improving tissue perfusion. The limbs should be kept warm as cold may precipitate pain.

The major aim of ulcer management is to remove necrotic tissue and to prevent infection. Selection of appropriate wound management products depends on the ulcer appearance, the amount of exudate and the position of the ulcer (see Section 4.2). The dressing needs to be effectively retained and yet not so bulky as to restrict mobility unduly. Some areas, such as the toes, are not at all easy to dress.

Bandages are often needed to hold the dressing in place. Compression bandages should not be used on arterial ulcers. Comfortable retention bandages such as cotton conforming bandages are suitable. Lightweight tubular bandages can be very useful, particularly on toes. It is important to ensure that, whatever bandage is used, it does not constrict the blood supply.

● *Evaluation* ●

The progress of both the patient and the ulcer should be evaluated. The effectiveness of pain control can be ascertained using a pain ruler (see Section 3.2.2). When monitoring the progress of the ulcer, attention should be paid to any indications of infection.

5.3.6 Ulcers of mixed aetiology

Some patients will have both an arterial and a venous component to their ulcer. It is important to define the predominant factor, so that appropriate treatment may be given.

● *Assessment* ●

Doppler assessment and assessment of the leg will provide an indication of the mixed aetiology. A full assessment in a vascular laboratory may be of benefit.

● *Planning* ●

If the main factor is venous, moderate graduated compression should be worn during the day. The degree of compression should be based on patient tolerance. Most patients will need to remove the compression garment at night when elevation of the legs is likely to increase ischaemic pain. When arterial disease predominates, compression may be impractical. However, exercise and short periods of limb elevation can be encouraged, within the limits of patient toleration.

● *Evaluation* ●

If healing is very slow, further advice from a vascular surgeon should be obtained.

5.3.7 Diabetic ulcers

Ulceration of the foot is a serious complication of diabetes mellitus. It is a major reason for the admission of people with diabetes to hospital in the UK (Young &

Boulton, 1991); in the USA, it is the cause of 50% of all non-traumatic amputations. The remaining leg becomes at considerable risk with 56% of patients undergoing amputation within five years (Levin, 1988). A full understanding of the aetiology and methods of prevention is essential to enable healthcare professionals to provide adequate education for the diabetics in their care.

Aetiology

The underlying causes of diabetic ulcers are peripheral neuropathy and peripheral vascular disease. Infection is an ever-present risk for the diabetic and can exacerbate the development of ulceration and increase the risk of amputation.

Peripheral neuropathy affects the peripheral sensory, motor and autonomic nerves of the leg. This has a two-fold effect of causing a loss of sensation and of compromising the biomechanics of the foot. Muscle atrophy in the foot, particularly over the arch of the foot, causes a transfer of body weight and reactive callus formation on the plantar surface. Ultimately, deformities of the foot, such as claw toes or Charcot foot, may occur together with alterations in gait. Walters *et al.* (1993) found foot ulceration was significantly associated with foot deformity. Poorly fitting shoes or a foreign body within the shoe can cause undetected injury resulting in ulcer formation. The patient may be completely unaware of the ulcer for some time.

Vascular disease in diabetics primarily affects the smaller arterioles within the foot. Intermittent claudication is unlikely as larger arteries are not usually occluded. Diabetic vascular disease is exacerbated by smoking. Gangrene of the toes can be caused by thrombosis in the artery supplying the affected digit. Pressure from poorly fitting shoes is the commonest cause of ischaemic ulceration.

Microvascular dilatation plays a significant role in the healing of minor wounds. The ability of these vessels to dilate can be measured by using a laser doppler to test the response to heat. A study by Sandeman *et al.* (1991) considered the ability to respond to heat by vasodilatation in insulin-dependent (ID) diabetics, non insulin-dependent (NID) diabetics and a control group of healthy individuals. A significantly worse response was found in the NID diabetics than in the other two groups.

Prevention

Given the grave implications of ulceration, prevention is very important. This can be achieved by patient education and adequate monitoring of the patient by the healthcare team. A multicentre study (Masson *et al.*, 1989) found that only 29% of 51 diabetic patients with new foot ulcers had previously considered that they were at risk of developing ulcers. Although many of the patients in the study were aware of the potential for foot problems, they did not consider themselves to be vulnerable. There is obviously need for improved patient education. Masson *et al.* (1989) suggest that this is best achieved by identifying the 'at-risk' groups and so targeting more specific educational strategies.

Young & Boulton (1991) have suggested guidelines for identifying those at risk of developing foot ulcers. They suggest that all new patients should be checked at the first visit to the diabetic clinic and then annually. Physical examination and screening by use of doppler ultrasound and quantative measures of nerve function should identify those at risk. Young & Boulton consider that patients with a history of previous ulceration, peripheral neuropathy, peripheral vascular disease, visual impairment, bony abnormalities, diabetic nephropathy or a history of alcohol abuse should all be considered to be at risk. So also should elderly patients or those who live alone.

Once a patient has been identified as being at risk, then she/he should be made aware of this and of her/his responsibilities for prevention of foot problems. Feet should be washed daily and dried carefully. They should be inspected for any red areas, swelling or cracked or broken skin. Toe nails should be cut straight across. Socks should be changed daily and not wrinkle. Shoes should be well fitting and checked for any foreign bodies before wearing. New shoes should be properly fitted and feet carefully observed for signs of rubbing. The patient should not wear sandals or go barefoot. Those with poor vision may need assistance. Those who smoke should stop.

At each attendance at the diabetic clinic, the patient should have a full foot check. This may involve the doctor, diabetic nurse specialist and chiropodist. Treatment of callus formation and management of any fungal infections is usually carried out by the chiropodist. If the patient has any deformity of the feet it may be helpful for the orthotist to assess her/him for suitable footwear. If the patient has other pathology requiring treatment, other health professionals should be vigilant in identifying any potential foot problems.

● *Assessment* ●

When assessing the patient there may be an indication of the type of ulcer. A history of pain associated with the ulcer, for example, almost certainly indicates ischaemia. Deformities of gait are indicative of neuropathy. Assessment of the diabetic state is important because of the increased risk of infection in the presence of hyperglycaemia.

Assessment of the leg and foot will provide objective evidence of the presence of either ischaemia or neuropathy or both. Table 5.4 indicates the differences between the two types of ulcers. However, both pathologies may be present in many patients. This mixed aetiology has been found in 40% of patients seen at a foot hospital (Young & Boulton, 1991). One aspect of assessment is to identify the precipitating factor; careful assessment of footwear and the precise position of the ulcer can provide clues. It is essential to identify the cause of the ulcer, or further ulceration may occur.

Neuropathic ulcers may be surrounded by callus and have a punched out appearance (see Plate 16). Ischaemic ulcers are usually covered by necrotic tissue. Neither type of ulcer has much exudate. The ulcer should be carefully observed for any indication of infection.

Wagner (1981) devised a scale for assessing diabetic ulcers, as follows:

Table 5.4   Comparison of signs of peripheral neuropathy and peripheral vascular disease in the diabetic foot.

Sign/symptom	Neuropathic ulcer	Ischaemic ulcer
Deformity of the foot:	Present as claw toe, hammer toe, Charcot foot or other.	Not present.
Skin temperature of foot:	Warm.	Cool.
Colour of foot:	Normal.	White when elevated or cyanotic.
Toe nails:	Atrophic.	Atrophic.
Pedal pulses:	Present.	Absent or diminished API is below 0.9.
Pain:	None.	Present, relieved by hanging legs down.
Callus formation:	Present, especially on plantar surface.	Not present.
Ulcer site:	Commonly on plantar surface of foot.	Commonly on toes and around the edges of the foot.

Grade 0   At-risk foot
Grade 1   Superficial ulcer, not clinically infected
Grade 2   Deeper ulcer, often infected, no osteomylitis
Grade 3   Deeper ulcer, abscess formation, osteomylitis
Grade 4   Localized gangrene (toe, forefoot or heel)
Grade 5   Gangrene of whole foot.

Ulcers graded 0–3 tend to be predominantly neuropathic, whereas in those graded 4 or 5 ischaemia is the main factor.

● *Planning* ●

Adequate control of the diabetic state is the primary goal when managing patients with foot ulceration. Pain control may also be necessary. Management of the ulcer depends on the causative factors. On the whole, neuropathic ulcers should be referred to the chiropodist as the callus needs to be removed before the ulcer can heal. Pressure must also be removed from the ulcer and this can be achieved by felt inserts, contact casting or even the use of crutches. Ischaemic ulcers may be resistant to treatment. Necrotic tissue must be debrided by use of appropriate wound management products. Any infection should be treated with systemic antibiotics and the application of suitable dressings (see Section 4.2). Compression bandages should not be used; if necessary, a simple retention bandage can be used to hold the dressing in place.

● *Evaluation* ●

Measurement of these ulcers by tracing may not provide adequate information as the surface area may not appear to alter greatly. A photographic record may be of more value. Careful assessment for any indication of infection should be made at each dressing change. Failure to respond to treatment can result in osteomyelitis. Surgical treatment is then necessary to eradicate the infection. Patients with ischaemic ulcers should be referred for a vascular consultation. Once the ulcer is healed, preventive measures need to be instigated.

Conclusions

Ulceration of the leg can cause untold suffering to the individual. Until recently little attention has been paid to the effect on a patient's lifestyle. A survey of 88 patients by Hamer *et al.* (1993) found that 37.5% felt that pain was the worst thing about having a leg ulcer. A further 30.7% complained of restriction of mobility. The majority of leg ulcer patients can be found in the community. Moffat *et al.* (1993) found that the use of community clinics with vascular support provided cost-effective care. Such clinics are cheaper than either individual visits by district nurses or visits to hospital outpatient departments. They also help to reduce patient isolation. Eagle (1992) highlights some of the benefits to both patients and nurses, in particular, the encouragement both feel as ulcers heal.

5.4 THE MANAGEMENT OF FUNGATING WOUNDS

Malignant fungating wounds are particularly difficult wounds to manage. They are distressing for both the sufferer and the nurse. A major problem is that there has been very little research into the management of this type of lesion. Most information seems to be anecdotal and nurses provide care based on previous experience or trial and error. Many of the patients with fungating wounds are cared for in the community. Whilst undoubtedly their nurses devote much time to caring for them, there is a need for research to be undertaken to improve the quality of life of these patients.

A recent postal survey (Thomas, 1992) has provided information about current practice in radiotherapy centres across the UK. Thomas noted that several respondants commented on the lack of published data and the generally unscientific approach to the management of fungating wounds.

5.4.1 Aetiology

Fungating lesions occur when a cancerous mass invades the epithelium, thus ulcerating through to the body surface. It most commonly occurs with cancer of the breast (Sims & Fitzgerald, 1985). However, it may also be found in cancers of the skin, vulva and bladder. Fungating wounds do not only develop at the site of the primary tumour; if the nodes of the groin or axilla are affected, ulceration may occur there also. Rosen (1980) suggests that almost any cancer may develop secondary deposits in the skin which can ulcerate.

Fungating lesions are often associated with neglect – that is, the patient delays seeking medical help. This is commonly seen in patients with breast cancers. A typical example is a lady who 'ignored' her breast lump for several years and only when her family noticed the offensive odour did she seek help.

5.4.2 Incidence

Little information seems to be available on this aspect of fungating wounds. Ivetic & Lyne (1990) have reviewed the literature and found no significant research. There seems to be some evidence that fungating lesions of the breast are less common than they once were, but it is not conclusive. The survey by Thomas (1992) found that breast lesions were most commonly seen, followed by head and neck lesions. However, the survey did not attempt to assess incidence.

5.4.3 Management of fungating wounds

Management of the patient

This is a vital part of the management of these wounds. Many factors within the patient can affect the progress of the wound. Chapter 3 discusses patient care in greater detail. Factors that need to be considered are:

Communication   the patient may find it too difficult to discuss his/her condition and its implications. Pain may also be a problem that needs to be addressed.

Eating and drinking   nutritional status may be affected by the disease process or by treatment such as radiotherapy or chemotherapy.

Elimination   poor nutrition may result in constipation. Some analgesia may also have the same effect. Ultimately, constipation will cause loss of appetite.

Mobility   poor mobility may affect the patient's ability to be self-caring.

Expressing sexuality   most patients are greatly distressed by their altered body image.

Sleeping   this may be disturbed because of anxiety and/or pain.

Dying   the prognosis for these patients is generally poor. The patient and his/her family are likely to need help in coming to terms with this.

Medical intervention   radiotherapy treatment may be given to reduce the size of the lesions and resolve some of the symptoms.

Psychological assessment   the patient may show signs of grief, fear or loss of self-respect. Some patients may talk of feeling 'unclean' or show embarrassment, especially when the wound is being dressed. Fitzgerald (Sims & Fitzgerald, 1985) describes how one lady talked of herself as 'leprous' and felt ashamed of her wound because it must be her fault. Patients who feel like this may not want others to dress their wound because they, the patients, believe that the wound would horrify them. *Spiritual assessment* the patient may question the meaning of life or express feelings of guilt and see the lesion as a form of punishment.

Management of the wound

Chapter 4 covers the general principles of wound management. This section will address the specific problems related to fungating wounds.

● *Assessment* ●

When assessing the wound the following need to be considered:

(1) Fungating lesions are often necrotic, sloughy or infected.
(2) There is usually copious amounts of exudate. It may have an offensive odour.
(3) Many of these wounds become malodorous as a result of bacterial invasion. This causes distress to the patient, relatives and visitors, and may be very difficult to control.
(4) The position of the wound obviously depends on the type of cancer. However, it may spread along the trunk or limbs, sometimes in the form of isolated nodules. Applying a dressing to protect such a spread out lesion can be very difficult and requires considerable nursing skill.
(5) Capillary bleeding may occur as the cancer increases in size and erodes blood vessels. This may be sufficiently heavy or frequent to cause anaemia. Removal of the old dressing must be done with great care in order to avoid loosening any clots.
(6) Lymphoedema may be present with cancers of the breast or vulva. This is a chronic swelling of the adjacent limb(s) due to a failure of lymph drainage. It may be associated with loss of function of the affected limb.

● *Planning* ●

It is essential to identify patient problems rather than nurse problems. Whilst in many instances they may be the same, they are not always. The following is an extreme example encountered by the author.

Mrs B. was admitted to hospital with a severely swollen leg due to lymphoedema. The ulceration in her groin was relatively small, but there was an ulcer on her leg which constantly poured lymph fluid. Despite being dressed by the district nurses three times a day, her leg was constantly wet and very painful. Initially, the problem of a painful wound was addressed by applying an extra absorbent hydrocolloid dressing. Within 48 hours, the pain had gone and Mrs B. looked a different person. The dressing was being changed daily. The nursing staff decided that the next problem to tackle was the lymphoedema, which would have the effect of reducing the fluid flowing from her leg. When Mrs B. was approached, she categorically said she was not interested. She wanted to go home as she had 'things to sort out' and she knew the district nurses would come and change her dressing when she needed them to do so. Mrs B. went home having had *her* problem resolved.

Once the specific problems have been identified, the treatment options have to be planned in the light of the patient's condition. If the expected outcome is very poor, then totally palliative care with the minimum need to dress the wound must be the treatment of choice. For others, a more aggressive approach can be used. A course of radiotherapy may be prescribed to help reduce the size of the lesion. It should be remembered that many patients find dressing change a major ordeal which leaves them feeling very tired.

Odour is probably the problem that provides the greatest distress to patients. It is mostly due to bacterial invasion, although exuding necrotic wounds may also be offensive. A wound swab will identify the offending bacteria so that appropriate systemic antibiotics can then be prescribed. Topical agents can also be used. Bower *et al.* (1992) found that metronidazole gel was effective in eliminating bacteria and reducing odour. Silver sulphadiazine cream can be used for *Pseudomonas aeruginosa* infections. Thomlinson (1980) cites the use of icing sugar on a fungating breast tumour as being effective in removing odour.

If the odour cannot be reduced, or even whilst action is being taken to reduce odour, other steps still can be investigated. The aim is to mask the smell, and this can be achieved in a variety of ways. Activated charcoal dressings can be effective in absorbing odour (Lawrence *et al.*, 1993). They are often used in conjunction with other dressings. Air fresheners can also help and stoma therapists can give advice on the use of deodorant solutions used by ostomists.

Copious exudate is another problem that concerns patients. Very absorbent dressings are necessary to provide patient comfort and dryness. Alginate dressings are probably the most effective, especially if the wound is necrotic or sloughy. Extra absorbent alginate dressings are available, reducing dressing change from many times a day to every 1–2 days. Some foam dressings are also very absorbent.

When aggressive treatment is suitable, wound debridement is a treatment option. Removal of necrotic or sloughy tissue can reduce odour and exudate. The quickest method is surgical debridement. This must be done by a skilled surgeon because of the distorted anatomy and the risk of capillary bleeding. Surgical debridement is not a suitable option for patients with a history of capillary bleeding into the wound. A variety of wound management products can be used, depending on the amount of exudate. Alginates and beads can be used on heavily exuding wounds. When there is moderate to low exudate, an amorphous hydrogel, enzymatic preparations and occasionally hydrocolloids can be used. The position, size and spread of the lesion can affect dressing choice.

Capillary bleeding can be frightening for both the patient and the nurse. When there is a history of capillary bleeding, great care should be taken when removing the old dressing. If the dressing is adherent, it should be well soaked with saline before removal is attempted. It may also be necessary to remove the dressing slowly in stages. It is better to take a long time to remove a dressing than to start bleeding which is difficult to control.

To control profuse bleeding, adrenaline can be applied directly to the wound.

However, it should be used with caution, and under medical supervision. Alginate dressings are useful when there is oozing. They can be removed easily by washing away with saline. If there is persistent bleeding, the patient's haemoglobin level should be checked regularly. Blood transfusions may be necessary to treat anaemia.

If radiotherapy treatment is being given to the lesion, attention must be given to dressing selection. The dressing must not contain any metal particles (such as zinc) as these will scatter the rays. A range of dressings have been found to be suitable: charcoal dressings, alginates and an amorphous hydrogel.

Dressing retention may be a problem. Ideally, the dressing should not be too bulky because it makes the wearing of clothes difficult and the patient becomes very self-conscious. Bandages and tubular net are probably the most versatile means of dressing retention. Tape should be used with care as the skin may become sore with repeated dressing change. If the patient is undergoing a course of radiotherapy to the lesion, it may be necessary for the outer dressing to be removed for treatment. Again, the skin may become sore. 'Garments' made from tubular net allow easy access to the wound and will not further damage the skin.

A novel method of providing a non-bulky and cosmetically pleasing dressing has been described by Grocott (1992). A fungating nodule on the angle of the neck and shoulder was successfully covered with a mould made from foamed latex. A keyhole allowed access to the nodule which was dressed with an alginate. Innovations such as this have quite a potential and further research is continuing. Collinson (1993) monitored the management of 350 patients over a four-year period. She devised protocols to improve the problems experienced by patients and carers, thus providing improved quality of life.

Patients with lymphoedema may have been told that nothing can be done to reduce the swelling. This is not true. Although it is not possible to *cure* lymphoedema, it can be controlled. It *is* possible to reduce a severely swollen limb to a reasonable size and so improve the quality of life of the patient (Badger, 1987). Management of lymphoedema involves a four-fold plan and considerable commitment from the patient and, possibly, a member of the family is needed. The aspects of care include compression, massage, exercise and skin care, and have been described by Badger & Twycross (1988).

Compression can be provided by bandages or compression hosiery, such as a sleeve. In the initial stages of treatment, bandages assist in reducing limb size. In severe cases, the digits as well as the hand and arm, or foot and leg should be bandaged. Once the limb has been reduced to a reasonable size, compression hosiery can then be used to maintain limb reduction.

Exercise assists in improving drainage of lymph from the limb. Muscle movement alters tissue pressure and has a massaging effect on the lymph vessels. The best effect is obtained if the exercises are carried out when the patient is wearing compression bandages or hosiery. Exercise also prevents or reduces stiffness of the joints. Passive movements should be carried out if the limb is paralysed. All patients should be encouraged to move as much as possible, but lifting and carrying heavy weights should be avoided.

Massage encourages the flow of lymph away from the limb. Occasionally, the swelling may have spread beyond the limb into the trunk. Massage should start on the trunk to clear lymph from the vessels there. This creates a space for the lymph in the swollen limb to flow into. The massage then continues down the affected limb. The massage technique should be gentle, so that it does not stimulate blood flow into the limb and increase congestion. It may need to be a little firmer when tissue fibrosis is present.

Intermittent pneumatic compression may be of use for some patients. It is used in addition to massage but is not an alternative. The type of compression that is most effective is the multichamber sequential pump. The best effect is obtained by clearing fluid from the trunk before commencing treatment.

Skin care is another vital aspect of care. Creams should be applied to prevent the skin drying out and cracking. Care should be taken to prevent the swollen limb getting burnt by the sun. Cuts and scratches can be a source of infection. They should be treated with antiseptic cream. Gloves should be worn for protection when working in the kitchen or garden. Jeffs (1993) has reviewed the effects of infection in lymphoedema. She suggests that *Streptococcus* is generally the causative organism. The infection should be treated with appropriate antibiotics.

It is important to provide encouragement to the patient to persevere with all aspects of this plan. None of these treatments is effective in isolation. Significant reduction of a swollen limb can only be achieved when all aspects of the treatment plan are implemented. Carroll & Rose (1992) demonstrated that this type of treatment regime reduced pain in the limb as well as limb volume. Williams (1993) described the benefits of a community-based lymphoedema service.

• *Evaluation* •

Evaluation of the management of fungating wounds should always consider whether the predetermined goals have been attained. Good documentation can be used to maintain a record of effective care, thus providing guidelines for the management of other patients. Managing a fungating wound and providing care for the patient require considerable nursing skills. More research is needed in order to be able to identify the most effective care.

REFERENCES

Allen, S. (1983) Hang the patient upside down from the ceiling – it works every time. *General Practitioner*, June 24, 40–41.

Audit Commission Review (1991) *The Virtue of Patients: Making the Best Use of Ward Nursing Resources*. The Audit Commission for Local Authorities and the National Health Service in England and Wales.

Badger, C. (1987) Lymphoedema: management of patients with advanced cancer. *Professional Nurse* **2**: 4, 100–2.

Badger, C. & Twycross, R. (1988) *Management of Lymphoedema*. Sir Michael Sobell House, Churchill Hospital, Oxford.

Baynes, V. (1984) Sore point in the NHS. *Nursing Mirror* **159**: 16, xi–xvi.

Bergstrom, N., Braden, B., Brandt, J. & Krall, K. (1985) Adequacy of descriptive scales for reporting diet intake in the institutionalised elderly. *Journal of Nutrition for the Elderly* **6**: 1, 3–16.

Bergstrom, N., Braden, B. & Laguzza, A. (1987) The Braden scale for predicting pressure sore risk. *Nursing Research* **36**: 4, 205–10.

Blair, S.D., Wright, D.D.I., Backhouse, C.M., Riddle, E. & McCollum, C.N. (1988) Sustained compression and healing of chronic leg ulcers. *British Medical Journal* **297**: 6657, 1159–61.

Bliss, M. (1990) (Editorial) Preventing pressure sores. *Lancet* **335**, 1311–12.

Bliss, M.R. & Thomas, J.M. (1993a) Clinical trials with budgetary implications: establishing randomised trials of pressure relieving aids. *Professional Nurse* **8**: 5, 292–6.

Bliss, M.R. & Thomas, J.M. (1993b) An investigative approach: an overview of randomised controlled trials of alternating pressure supports. *Professional Nurse* **8**: 7, 437–44.

Bliss, M.R. & Thomas, J.M. (1993c) Making sense of comparative values: evaluation of trials of constant low pressure supports. *Professional Nurse* **8**: 9, 564–70.

Bosanquet, N. (1992) Costs of venous ulcers: from maintenance therapy to investment programmes. *Phlebology* **7**: 1, 44–46.

Bower, M., Stein, R., Evans, T.R.J., Hedley, A., Pert, P. & Coombes, R.C. (1992) The double-blind study of the efficacy of metronidazole gel in the treatment of malodorous fungating tumours. *European Journal of Cancer* **28a**: 45, 888–9.

Bridel, J. (1993) Pressure sore risk in operating theatres. *Nursing Standard* **7**: 32, suppl. 4–10.

Burnand, K. (1988) Fibrin and fibrinolysis in ulceration. In Cederholm-Williams, S.A., Ryan, T.J. & Lydon, M.J. (eds) *Fibrinolysis and Angiogenesis in Wound Healing.* Excerpta Medica, Princeton.

Callam, M.J., Ruckley, C.V., Harper, D.R. & Dale, J.J. (1985) Chronic ulceration of the leg: extent of the problems and provision of care. *British Medical Journal* **290**: 1855–6.

Cameron, J. (1990) Patch-testing for leg ulcer patients. *Nursing Times* **86**: 25, 63–4.

Cameron, J. (1991) Compression therapy. *Primary Health Care* **1**: 7, 14–18.

Carroll, D. & Rose, K. (1992) Treatment leads to significant improvement: effects of conservative treatment on pain in lymphoedema. *Professional Nurse* **8**: 1, 32–36.

Chapman, E.J. & Chapman, R. (1986) Treatment of pressure sores: the state of the art. In Tierney, A.J. (ed) *Clinical Nursing Practice*, Churchill Livingstone, Edinburgh.

Clark, O., Barbanel, J.C., Jordan, M.M. & Nicol, M. (1978) Pressure sores. *Nursing Times* **74**: 9, 363–6.

Clark, M. & Cullum, N. (1992) Matching patient need for pressure sore prevention with the supply of pressure redistributing mattresses. *Journal of Advanced Nursing* **17**, 310–16.

Colgan, M.P., Dormandy, J.A., Jones, P.W. *et al.* (1990) Oxypentifylline treatment of venous ulcers of the leg. *British Medical Journal* **300**, 972–5.

Collinson, G. (1993) Improving the quality of life in patients with malignant fungating wounds. In Harding, K.G., Cherry, G., Dealey, C. & Turner, T.D. (eds) *Proceedings of the 2nd European Conference on Advances in Wound Management*, Macmillan Magazines, London.

Cornwall, J.V., Dore, C.J. & Lewis, J.D. (1986) Leg ulcers: epidemiology and aetiology. *British Medical Journal* **73**: 693–6.

Cullum, N. & Clark, M. (1992) Intrinsic factors associated with pressure sores in elderly people. *Journal of Advanced Nursing* **17**, 427–31.

Dale, J. & Gibson, B. (1986) Leg ulcers: a disease affecting all ages. *Professional Nurse* **1**: 8, 213–17.

Dale, J. & Gibson, B. (1990) Back-up for the venous pump. *Professional Nurse* **5**: 9, 481–86.

David, J.A., Chapman, R.G., Chapman, E.J. & Lockett, B. (1983) An investigation of the current methods used in nursing for the care of patients with established pressure sores. Nursing Practice Research Unit, Nothwick Park, Middlesex.

Dealey, C. (1989a) The pressure sore debate. *Nursing Times* **85**: 26, 75.

Dealey, C. (1989b) The specialist in tissue viability. *Nursing* **4**: 1, 16–19.

Dealey, C. (1990) How are you supporting your patients? *Professional Nurse* **6**: 3, 134–41.

Dealey, C. (1991a) The size of the pressure sore problem in a teaching hospital. *Journal of Advanced Nursing* **16**, 663–70.

Dealey, C. (1991b) Causes of leg ulcers. *Nursing* **4**: 35, 23–24.

Dealey, C. (1992) Pressure sores; the result of bad nursing? *British Journal of Nursing* **1**: 15, 748.

Dealey, C., Earwaker, T. & Eden, L. (1991) Are your patients sitting comfortably? *Journal of Tissue Viability* **1**: 2, 36–39.

Dealey, C. (1993) Pressure sores: the result of bad nursing? *British Journal of Nursing* **1**: 15, 748.

Department of Health (1992) *Health of the Nation.* HMSO, London.

Durham, M. & Grice, A. (1991) Unhealthy British lifestyle is killing the sick man of Europe. *Sunday Times* no. 8702, 2nd June, 2.

Eagle, M. (1992) Community clinics. *Nursing Times* **88**: 46, 61–4.

Eaglestein, W.H., Falanga, V., Nemeth, A. & Moosa, H. (1988) Pericapillary fibrin, venous ulcers and transcutaneous oxygen. In Cederholm-Williams, S.A. Ryan, T.J., Lyden, M.J. (eds) *Fibrinolysis and Angiogenesis in Wound Healing*, Excerpta Medica, Princeton.

Ek, A.C. & Boman, G. (1982) A descriptive study of pressure sores: the prevalence of pressure sores and the characteristics of patients. *Journal of Advanced Nursing* **7**, 51–57.

Ek, A.C. Gustavssen, G. & Lewis, D.H. (1987) Skin blood flow in relation to external pressure and temperature in the supine position on a standard hospital mattress. *Scandinavian Journal of Rehabilitation* **19**: 121–6.

Exton-Smith, A.N. & Shermin, R.W. (1961) The prevention of pressure sores: the significance of spontaneous bodily movement. *Lancet* **II**, 1124–26.

Fentem, P.H. (1986) Elastic hosiery. *Pharmacy Update* **5**, 200–205.

Flanagan, M. (1993) Pressure sore risk assessment scales. *Journal of Wound Care* **2**: 3, 162–7.

Fowler, E. (1990) Chronic wounds: an overview. In Krasner, D. (ed) *Chronic Wound Care: A Clinical Sourcebook for Healthcare Professionals.* Health Management Publications Inc., King of Prussia, Pennsylvania.

General, Municipal and Boilermakers Union (1985) *Hazard in the Health Service – An A–Z guide.* GMB, London.

Gilchrist, B. (1998) Treating leg ulcers. *Nursing Times, Community Outlook* **85**: 6, suppl. 25–26.

Goldstone, L.A. & Goldstone, J. (1982) The Norton Score: an early warning of pressure sores. *Journal of Advanced Nursing* **7**, 419–26.

Grocott, P. (1992) The latest on latex. *Nursing Times* **88**: 12, suppl. 1–2.

Hamer, C., Cullum, N. & Roe, B.H. (1993) Patients' perceptions of chronic leg ulceration. In Harding, K.G., Cherry, G., Dealey, C. & Turner, T.D. (eds) *Proceedings of 2nd European Conference in Advances in Wound Management.* Macmillan Magazines Ltd., London.

Harkiss, K.J. (1985) Cost analysis of dressing materials used in venous leg ulcers. *Pharmaceutical Journal* **235**: 6344, 268–69.

Health and Safety Executive (1992) *Manual Handling: Manual Handling Operations Regulations. Guidance on Regulations.* HSE, London.

Hibbs, P. (1988) Pressure area care for the City and Hackney Health Authority. City and Hackney Health Authority, London.

Hibbs, P. (1990) The economics of pressure sore prevention. In Border, D. (ed) *Pressure Sores – Clinical Practice and Scientific Approach.* Macmillan Press Ltd., London.

Ivetic, O. & Lyne, P.A. (1990) Fungating and ulcerating malignant lesions: a review of the literature. *Journal of Advanced Nursing* **15**, 83–8.

Jeffs, E. (1993) The effect of acute inflammatory episodes on the treatment of lymphoedema. *Journal of Tissue Viability* **3**: 2, 51–5.

Jordan, M.M. & Clark, M. (1977) Report on incidence of pressure sores in the patient community of the Greater Glasgow Health Board area. University of Strathclyde, Glasgow, Jan. 21.

Khoo, C. & Bailey, B.N. (1990) Reconstructive surgery. In Bader, D. (ed) *Pressure Sores – Clinical Practice and Scientific Approach.* MacMillan Press, London.

Klazinga, N. & Geibing, H. (1993) Prevention of pressure sores as a topic for quality assurance. Results of the first phase of a European Concerted Action Programme. In Harding, K.G., Cherry, G., Dealey, C. & Turner, T.D. (eds) *Proceedings of the 2nd European Conference on Advances in Wound Management.* Macmillan Magazines Ltd, London.

Krasner, D. (1990) Pressure ulcers: an overview. In Krasner, D. (ed) *Chronic Wound Care: a Clinical Sourcebook for Healthcare Professionals.* Health Management Publications Inc., King of Prussia, Pennsylvania.

Krouskop, M. (1983) A synthesis of the factors which contribute to pressure sore formation. *Medical Hypothesis* **11**, 255–67.

Kulkarni, J. & Philbin, M. (1993) Pressure sore awareness survey in a university teaching hospital. *Journal of Tissue Viability* **3**: 3, 77–9.

Landis, E.M. (1931) Micro-injection studies of capillary blood pressure in human skin. *Heart* **15**, 209–28.

Lawrence, J.C., Lilly, H.A. & Kidson, A. (1993) Malodour and dressings containing active charcoal. In Harding K.G., Cherry, G., Dealey, C. & Turner, T.d. (eds) *Proceedings of the 2nd European Conference on Advances in Wound Management.* Macmillan Magazines Ltd., London.

Levin, M.E. (1988) The diabetic foot: pathophysiology evaluation and treatment. In Levin, M.E. & O'Neal, L.W. (eds) *The Diabetic Foot* (4th edn). C.V. Mosby, St Louis.

Livesley, B. & Simpson, G. (1989) The hard cost of soft sores. *Health Service Journal* **99**: 5138, 231.

Livesley, B. & Simpson, G. (1993) *Prevention and Management of Pressure Sores within Hospital and Community Settings.* Research for Ageing Trust, London.

Lockett, B. (1983) Prevalence and incidence. In *Symposium on Pressure Sore Disease.* Royal Hospital and Home for Incurables, London.

Logan, R.A., Thomas, S., Harding, E.F. & Collyer, G.J. (1992) A comparison of sub-bandage pressure produced by experienced and inexperienced bandagers. *Journal of Wound Care* **1**: 3, 23–5.

Loudon, I.S.L. (1982) Leg ulcers in the eighteenth and early nineteenth centuries. *Journal of the Royal College of General Practitioners* **32**, 301–9.

Lowthian, P. (1979) Turning clocks, a system to prevent pressure sores. *Nursing Mirror* **148**: 21, 30–31.

Lowthian, P. (1987a) The practical assessment of pressure sore risk. *Care – Science and Practice* **5**: 4, 3–7.

Lowthian, P. (1987b) The classification and grading of pressure sores. *Care – Science and Practice* **5**: 1, 5–9.

Lowthian, P. (1989) Pressure sore prevention. *Nursing* **3**: 34, 17–23.

Magazinovic, N., Phillips-Turner, J. & Wilson, G.V. (1993) Assessing nurses' knowledge of bandages and bandaging. *Journal of Wound Care* **2**: 2, 97–101.

Masson, E.A., Angle, S., Roseman, P., Soper, C., Wilson, I., Cotton, M. & Boulton, A.J.M. (1989) Diabetic ulcers – do patients know how to protect themselves. *Practical Diabetes* **6**: 1, 22–3.

Mayberry, J.C., Moneta, G.L., Taylor, L.M. & Porter, J.M. (1991) Fifteen-year results of ambulatory compression therapy for chronic venous ulcers. *Surgery* **109**: 5, 575–81.

McClement, E.J.W. (1984) No pressure – no sore. *Journal of Nursing* **2**: 21, suppl. 1–3.

Milward, P. (1988) Personal Communication, Walsall Health Authority.

Milward, P. (1993) How to manage pressure sores in the community. *British Journal of Nursing* **2**: 9, 488–92.

Moffat, C.J. & Dickson, D. (1993) The Charing Cross high compression four-layer bandage system. *Journal of Wound Care* **2**: 2, 91–4.

Moffatt, C.J., Franks, P.J., Oldroyd, M. & Greenhalgh, R.M. (1993) Evaluation of community leg ulcer clinics. In Harding, K.G., Cherry, G., Dealey, C., Turner, T.D. (eds) *Proceedings of 2nd European Conference on Advances in Wound Management*. Macmillan Magazines Ltd., London.

Mulder, G., Robison, J. & Seeley, J. (1990) Study of sequential compression therapy in the treatment of non-healing chronic venous ulcers. *Wounds* **2**: 3, 111–15.

National Pressure Ulcer Advisory Panel (1989) Pressure ulcers incidence, economics and risk assessment. *Care – Science and Practice* **7**: 4, 96–99.

Negus, D. & Friedgood, A. (1983) The effective management of venous ulceration. *British Journal of Surgery* **70**: 10, 623–7.

Nightingale, F. (1861) *Notes on Nursing*. Appleton Century, New York.

Norton, D., Exton-Smith, A.N. & Mclaren, R. (1975) *An Investigation of Geriatic Nursing Problems in Hospital*. Churchill Livingstone, Edinburgh.

Nyquist, R. & Hawthorn, P.J. (1987) The prevalence of pressure sores in an area health authority. *Journal of Advanced Nursing* **12**, 183–7.

Nyquist, R. & Hawthorn, P.J. (1988) The incidence of pressure sores amongst a group of elderly patients with fractured neck of femur. *Care – Science and Practice* **6**: 1, 3–7.

O'Dea, K. (1993) Prevalence of pressure damage in hospital patients in the UK. *Journal of Wound Care* **2**: 4, 221–5.

Pinchcofski-Devin, G. & Kaminski, M.V. (1986) Correlation of pressure sores and nutritional status. *Journal of the American Geriatic Society* **34**, 435–40.

Podmore, J. (1993) Report on Tissue Viability Society Spring Conference. *Nursing Standard* **7**: 32, suppl. 14.

Preston, K.W. (1988) Positioning for comfort and pressure relief: the 30 degree alternative. *Care – Science and Practice* **6**: 4, 116–9.

Preston, K. (1991) Counting the cost of pressure sores. *Community Outlook* **1**: 9, 19–24.

Pritchard, V. (1986) Calculating the risk. *Nursing Times* **82**: 8, 59–61.

Rithalia, S.V.S. (1989) Comparison of pressure distribution in wheelchair seat cushions. *Care – Science and Practice* **7**: 4, 87–9.

Robertson, J., Swain, I. & Gaywood, I. (1990) The importance of pressure sores in total health care. In Bader, O. (ed) *Pressure Sores – Clinical Practice and Scientific Approach*. Macmillan Press, London.

Rosen, T. (1980) Cutaneous metastases. *Medical Clinics of North America* **64**: 5, 885–900.

Royal College of Physicians (1986) Physical disability in 1986 and beyond. *Journal of the Royal College of Physicians of London* **20**: 3, 160–94.

Ryan, T.J. (1987) *The Management of Leg Ulcers* (2nd ed.). Oxford University Press, Oxford.

Sandeman, D.D., Pym, C.A., Green, E.M., *et al.* (1991) Microvascular vasodilation in the feet of newly diagnosed non-insulin dependent diabetics. *British Medical Journal* **302**: 6785, 1122–3.

Schraibman, I.G. (1987) The bacteriology of leg ulcers. *Phlebology* **2**: 4, 265–9.

Sims, R. & Fitzgerald, V. (1985) *Community Nursing Management of Patients with Ulcerating/Fungating Breast Disease.* Royal College of Nursing, London.

Stemmer, R. (1969) Ambulatory elasto-compressive treatment of the lower extremities particularly with elastic stockings. *Der Kassenatzt* **9**, 1–8.

Thomas, S. (1990a) Cost-effective management of leg ulcers. *Nursing Times, Community Outlook* **86**: 11, suppl. 21–22.

Thomas, S. (1990b) Bandages and bandaging. *Nursing Standard* **4**: 39, suppl. 4–6.

Thomas, S. (1992) *Current Practices in the Management of Fungating Lesions and Radiation Damaged Skin.* Surgical Materials Testing Laboratory, Bridgend, Glamorgan.

Thomlinson, R.H. (1980) Kitchen remedy for necrotic malignant breast ulcers. *Lancet* 8196, 707.

Torrance, C. (1983) *Pressure Sores: Aetiology, Treatment and Prevention.* Croom Helm, London.

United Kingdom Central Council for Nursing, Midwifery and Health Visiting (UKCC) (1992) *Code of Professional Conduct for the Nurse, Midwife and Health Visitor.* UKCC, London.

United States' Department of Health and Human Services (1992) Pressure ulcers in adults: prediction and prevention. Quick reference guide for clinicians. *Decubitus* **5**: 3, 26–30.

United States' Department of Health and Human Services (1992) Preventing pressure ulcers: a patient's guide. *Decubitus* **5**: 3, 34–40.

Versluysen, M. (1986) How elderly patients with femoral fractures develop pressure sores in hospital. *British Medical Journal* **292**, 1311–13.

Wagner, F.W. (1981) The dysvascular foot: a system for diagnosis and treatment. *Foot Ankle* **2**, 64.

Walters, D.P., Gatling, W., Hill, R.D. & Mullee, M.A. (1993) The prevalence of foot deformity in diabetic subjects: a population study in an English community. *Practical Diabetes* **10**: 3, 106–8.

Warner, U. & Hall, D.J. (1986) Pressure sores: a policy for prevention. *Nursing Times* **82**: 6, 59–61.

Waterlow, J. (1985) A risk assessment card. *Nursing Times* **81**: 48, 49–55.

Waterlow, J. (1988) Prevention is cheaper than cure. *Nursing Times* **84**: 25, 69–70.

Williams, A. (1993) Management of lymphoedema: a community-based approach. *British Journal of Nursing* **2**: 13, 678–81.

Young, J. (1992) The use of specialised beds and mattresses. *Journal of Tissue Viability* **2**: 3, 79–81.

Young, J. (1993) Pressure sores and the quality of care: a report on a joint Department of Health and Clinical Standards Advisory Group conference, London, May 1993. *Journal of Tissue Viability* **3**: 3, 72–73.

Young, M.J. & Boulton, A.J.M. (1991) Guidelines for identifying the at-risk foot. *Practical Diabetes* **8**: 3, 103–5.

Chapter 6
The Management of Patients with Acute Wounds

6.1 INTRODUCTION

Acute wounds can be defined as wounds of sudden onset and of short duration. They include surgical wounds and traumatic wounds such as burns. Acute wounds can occur in people of all ages and generally heal easily without complication. This chapter will consider the specific care needed for patients with acute wounds.

6.2 THE CARE OF SURGICAL WOUNDS

Surgical wounds are, by their very nature, premeditated wounds. This allows the surgeon to attempt to reduce any risks of complication to a minimum. However, as increasingly sophisticated surgery is performed, often on relatively elderly patients, complications are still a hazard. One aspect of nursing care is to monitor the progress of the wound, so that there is an early identification of any problems.

6.2.1 Management of surgical wounds

● *Patient assessment* ●

This is essential to identify any factors that can affect healing. This topic is covered in more detail in Chapter 3. Potential problem areas include:

Maintaining a safe environment   the risk of infection must be considered.
Communicating   identify patient understanding of the operative procedure. Postoperative pain must be assessed and controlled.
Breathing   recording of vital signs for indication of haemorrhage.
Eating and drinking   assessment of nutritional status is essential as patients may be starved for long periods.
Controlling body temperature   pyrexia is an indication of infection.
Mobilizing   mobility is often reduced in the postoperative period.
Expressing sexuality   assess the patient's reaction to his/her altered body image.
Sleeping   sleeping patterns may be altered because of pain and/or disturbance by nursing staff.
Psychological care   particular problems which may be identified are fear and powerlessness.
Spiritual care   spiritual distress may be caused by loss of meaning or purpose in life.

● *Wound assessment* ●

This should identify the method of closure, note the use of any drains and observe for any indication of complication.

Westaby (1985) describes the main aim of surgical wound closure as being the restoration of function and physical integrity with the minimum deformity and without infection. The method of wound closure is selected in order to achieve this aim and it will vary according to the surgery performed. There are three methods of closure: primary closure, delayed primary closure, and healing by second intention.

Primary closure

Hippocrates (460–377 BC) was the first to describe this method of wound closure. He called it healing by first intention. The skin edges are held in approximation by sutures, clips, staples or tape. In these wounds the skin edges seal very quickly – first with fibrin from clot formation and then as epithelialization occurs. Within 48 hours the wound should be totally sealed, thus preventing the ingress of bacteria.

Delayed primary closure

This method of closure is used when there has been considerable bacterial contamination. Initially, any body cavity is closed and the remaining tissue layers are left open to allow free drainage of pus. After about five days, these layers are closed and the wound will heal as any primarily closed wound. Wound drains may be used to assist in the removal of any fluid remaining at the wound base.

Healing by second intention

Healing by second intention describes a wound that is left open and heals by granulation, contraction and epithelialization. This method may be used for a variety of reasons. For example:

(a)   There may be considerable tissue loss, e.g. radical vulvectomy.
(b)   The surgical incision is shallow, but has a large surface area, e.g. donor sites.
(c)   There may have been infection (for example, a ruptured appendix) or an abscess may have been drained, and free drainage of any pus is essential.

Wound drains

Wound drains are inserted to provide a channel to the body surface for fluid which might otherwise collect in the wound. The fluid may be blood, pus, serous exudate, bile or other body fluids. There are several different types of drains (see Fig. 6.1). Torrance (1993) has described them in some detail. They can be divided into open and closed drains.

Closed drains consist of the drain, connection tubing and the collecting receptacle. They usually provide a vacuum and so have a suction effect.

Chest drains are closed drains which work rather differently. The purpose of this

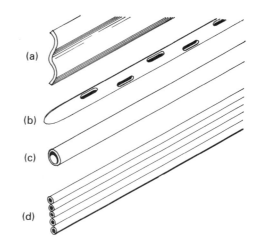

(a)

(b)

(c)

(d)

Fig. 6.1   Different types of wound drains:
(a) sump or corrugated drain; (b) drain for
closed system with multiple perforations;
(c) Penrose drain; (d) Yeats drain.

type of system is to allow air to escape from the cavity and bubble into the water in the container.

Open drains may be tubes, corrugated rubber or plastic, or soft tubes filled with ribbon gauze to provide a wicking effect. Open drains originally drained into the dressing, causing considerable discomfort to the patient. They also increased the risk of infection as the drain provided an open channel for bacteria. However, drainage bags are now available to cover the drain, thus simulating a closed circuit.

Closed drains are usually inserted through a stab wound adjacent to the incision. Open drains may either be inserted through a similar stab wound or drain from the wound itself.

Cruse & Foord (1973; 1980) considered the effect of wound drains on infection rates for the surgical wound. Of particular interest was the use of drains with cholecystectomy. They found the following infection rates:

closed suction drain   0% infection rate
stab drain   1.8% infection rate
no drain   2.9% infection rate
drain through wound   9.9% infection rate

The use of drains is essential to prevent the collection of fluid in the wound, but the position of a drain may actually increase the risk of infection rather than reduce it. However, since the results of Cruse & Foord's (and similar) studies have been published, the practice of placing drains through the wound has considerably diminished.

Potential complications following surgery

A variety of complications may occur following surgery. Only those related to the wound will be discussed here.

Haemorrhage   Severe blood loss may occur during surgery, in the immediate postoperative period and up to ten days afterwards. This is sometimes referred to as primary, intermediary and secondary haemorrhage. The main cause of both primary and intermediary haemorrhage is poor surgical technique. This is either due to failure to control bleeding during surgery, or to poorly tied blood vessels. As the blood pressure returns to normal levels the clots and ties get pushed off the end of the blood vessel(s) resulting in bleeding. Secondary haemorrhage is invariably associated with infection.

Taylor et al. (1987) studied the effects of haemorrhage on wound strength. They found that perioperative bleeding caused a weaker suture line which was associated with impaired fibroblast function. The researchers suggest that non-absorbable or long lasting sutures should be used if haemorrhage occurs during surgery.

The bleeding may be brisk and rapidly seen, or it may be more insidious. Blood may be seen on the wound dressing or it may drain into a drainage bag. If the bleeding is internal, signs of shock may be the first indication of loss of blood. If there is only a little bleeding, the blood may ooze into the superficial tissues and show as bruising around the suture line. Slow seepage of blood may lead to haematoma formation when the blood collects in a 'dead space' around the operative site and then clots.

If there is heavy bleeding, further surgery may be needed to find and control the bleeding point. In many cases the bleeding is monitored closely to see if further clotting will resolve the problem. When a haematoma forms it is a potential breeding ground for bacteria. It is sometimes possible to remove a suture in order to evacuate the haematoma.

Infection   Despite considerable improvement in standards of asepsis, post-surgical wound infection still occurs. Measuring infection rates is one method used in evaluating standards of care for surgical audit. Overall infection rates of 4.7% (Cruse & Foord, 1980), 5.4% (Leigh, 1981) and 7.3% (Mishriki et al., 1990) were found in surveys of the incidence of surgical wound infection. It is not possible to make direct comparisons between these surveys because the criteria for defining wound infection varies. Cruse & Foord, for example, used the following definition: 'a wound is defined as infected if it discharges pus'. A recent study by Bell & Fenton (1993) highlights the importance of continuing infection surveillance after discharge from hospital. This is particularly relevant for day surgery patients and those discharged early from hospital.

Mishriki et al. (1990) described the variety of ways used to define surgical wound infection and the need for more conformity. Wilson et al. (1990) have addressed this problem and have produced a scoring system which they found to be reproducible. The ASEPSIS wound scoring system, with the grading for the severity of infection, is shown in Fig. 6.2. The authors compared this system with other methods when assessing 1029 surgical patients. They suggest that it is particularly suitable for use in clinical trials, but would need to be modified for surgical audit. Bibby et al. (1986) suggested a different model for auditing wound infection. Their model mathematically predicts the likelihood of wound infection in individual patients. This information can then be compared with the actual outcome. Over time, this would provide information about the performance of different surgeons.

When measuring the incidence of surgical wound infections it is essential to

TABLE A

Wound characteristic	Proportion of wound affected (%)					
	0	< 20	20–29	40–59	60–79	> 80
Serous exudate	0	1	2	3	4	5
Erythema	0	1	2	3	4	5
Purulent exudate	0	2	4	6	8	10
Separation of deep tissues	0	2	4	6	8·	10

TABLE B

Criteria for allocation of additional points to ASEPSIS Score

Criterion	Points
Additional treatment:	
Antibiotics	10
Drainage of pus under local anaesthetic	5
Debridement of wound (general anaesthetic)	10
Serous discharge	daily 0–5
Erythema	daily 0–5
Purulent drainage	daily 0–10
Separation of deep tissues	daily 0–10
Isolation of bacteria	10
Stay as inpatient prolonged over 14 days	5

Score **Table A** daily for first week, add points from **Table B** for any criteria satisfied in first 2 months after surgery.

Category of infection: total score 0–10 = satisfactory healing, 11–20 = disturbance of healing; 21–30 = minor wound infection; 31–40 = moderate wound infection; > 40 = major wound infection.

Fig. 6.2 The ASEPSIS wound score.

(From: Wilson, A.P.R., Weavill, C., Burridge, J., & Kelsey, M.C. (1990).)
Reproduced with permission of Academic Press Ltd.

understand the potential causes. The causes of infection can be divided into factors related to the environment, the patient and the surgery, and are summarized in Table 6.1. The first two factors have already been discussed in Section 3.2. Factors relating to the surgery need to be considered. One of the most important factors is the type of surgery being undertaken. Cruse & Foord (1973; 1980) used a method of categorizing types of surgery which has since become widely recognized and used in other studies. Their categories of operations are: (1) clean, (2) clean-contaminated, (3) contaminated, and (4) dirty. Table 6.2 explains these categories

Table 6.1 Factors increasing the incidence of surgical wound infection.

Environment

Lengthy preoperative hospitalization
High bed occupancy
Poor standards of asepsis within the theatre suite
Unsuitable layout within the theatre suite
Inadequate ventilation in operating theatre

Patient

Age
Obesity
Malnutrition
Diabetes
Steroids
Immunosuppressive drugs
Additional lesions, e.g. pressure sore (form reservoir of bacteria)
Shaving

Wound

Type of surgery
Length of surgery
Time of surgery
Poor surgical technique
Position of drains

Based on Dealey, C. (1991).

and shows the infection rates found by Cruse & Foord (1980). There is a dramatic difference in infection rates between clean and dirty surgery. The clean wound infection rate is usually used as a baseline for monitoring other factors which may affect infection rates. Richold (1992) also found different infection rates in different specialities with clean wound infection rates of 2.0% in general surgery, 2.9% in orthopaedics, 5.2% in obstetrics and 6.6% following Caesarian section.

Probably the most important factor to consider is surgical technique. Cruse & Foord (1980) found that meticulous attention to detail was essential to keep clean wound infection rates low. They also noted that informing staff of all cases of wound infection and providing surgeons with details of *their* infection rates and that of their colleagues, helped to reduce clean wound infection rates. A more recent study by Mishriki *et al.* (1990) supports this view. They found a strong association between the individual surgeon and the development of infection. The elimination of one surgeon's case-load would have reduced the clean wound infection rate by over 40%. Mishriki *et al.* suggest that in-house surgical audit and peer review should be a fundamental aspect of quality assurance.

Other factors which have been shown to have some relevance to the development of infection include the length of operations. Cruse & Foord (1980) found that the clean wound infection rate doubled for every hour of surgery. They suggest four possible reasons for this increase: (1) wound cells are damaged by drying out when exposed to air; (2) the total amount of bacterial contamination increases with time;

Table 6.2   Classification of surgical wounds.

Clean
Surgery where there was no infection seen, no break in asepsis and hollow muscular organs not entered. Could include hysterectomy, cholecystectomy, or appendicectomy 'in passing' if no evidence of inflammation.
Infection rate: 1.5%

Clean-contaminated
Where a hollow muscular organ entered, but only minimal spillage of contents.
Infection rate: 7.7%

Contaminated
When a hollow viscus was opened with gross spillage of contents, acute inflammation without pus found, a major break in asepsis or traumatic wounds less than four hours old.
Infection rate: 15.2%

Dirty
Traumatic wounds more than four hours old. Surgery where a perforated viscus or pus is found.
Infection rate: 40%

(Based on Cruse, P.J.E. & Foord, R. (1980).)

(3) the longer the operation, the more sutures and electrocoagulation are used; (4) longer surgery may be associated with shock and/or blood loss, thus reducing resistance to infection. Although it is not possible to eliminate all these factors, the numbers of bacteria in the air can be reduced. Air filtration systems can be used, but Cruse & Foord suggested that the same results would be obtained by some fairly simple measures, such as: reducing conversation and the amount of movement in and out of the theatre, and excluding anyone with any skin infection.

The timing of surgery also affects infection rates. Cruse & Foord (1980) found that when clean and clean-contaminated surgery was carried out at night-time there was almost double the infection rate of that in the day. This is most likely to be due to weariness in the surgical team leading to imperfect surgical technique.

Dehiscence   Dehiscence means the breaking down, or splitting open, of all or part of a wound healing by first intention. It is most frequently seen in abdominal wounds (Westaby, 1985). Complete dehiscence may involve evisceration of the gut – or 'burst abdomen'. If the skin remains intact when the muscle and fascia layers break down, an incisional hernia occurs – which may not necessarily become obvious for some months following surgery.

Dehiscence can occur because of systemic and local factors. Poole (1985) reviewed clinical reports of abdominal dehiscence between 1950 and 1984. He noted that several systemic factors had been identified – malnutrition, age, male sex and long term use of steroids. Poole suggests that these factors are overstated and that local factors have a much greater significance. In particular, he considered wound infection, abdominal distension and pulmonary complications the most important. One example is a prospective study of 1129 major laparotomies carried out by Bucknall *et al.* (1982) where all patients were followed up for a year after surgery. There were 1.7% burst abdomens and 7.4% incisional hernias. The incidence of herniation was compared with a variety of factors. Whilst obesity, age and male sex were found to be of significance, the presence of wound infection, chest infection and abdominal distension were all highly significant. The method of wound closure was also of importance: mass closure was found to reduce the incidence of burst abdomen from 3.8% to 0.8%.

Westaby (1985) considers that surgical technique may be a factor in dehiscence. Securing sutures too tightly so that the sutures cut into the tissues can result in dehiscence. Tight suturing also affects the vascularity of the skin edges, with areas of necrosis around the sutures. Occasionally, failure of the suture material may occur. This is less common with non-absorbable sutures. Perkins (1992) suggests that dehiscence can be divided into early wound dehiscence and late wound dehiscence. She suggests that early dehiscence is related to suture failure and/or surgical technique and that late dehiscence is more likely to be the result of infection.

Sinus formation   A sinus is a track to the body surface from an abscess or some material which is an irritant and becomes a focus for infection. A common irritant is suture material. Dressing material, such as ribbon gauze may also be retained and prevent healing. Sinuses can become chronic if the causative factor is not resolved. A sinogram will show the extent of a sinus and help to identify the root problem. Surgical excision or laying open of the sinus is usually the most effective form of management. Once the focus for infection has been removed and free drainage can occur, the remaining cavity will heal by granulation and contraction.

Fistula formation   A fistula is an abnormal track connecting one viscus with another viscus, or connecting a viscus with the body surface. They may develop spontaneously or following surgery. Common examples are: rectovaginal (connecting the rectum and vagina), biliary (allowing leakage of bile to the surface following surgery on the gall bladder and/or bile ducts); faecal (allowing leakage of faecal fluid through the wound, often associated with infection). Persistent leakage of fluid indicates the possible presence of a fistula. Examination of the fluid will usually indicate the source of the fistula.

The majority of fistulae will close spontaneously. Conservative treatment to maintain the integrity of the skin and the nutritional status of the patient is the treatment of choice, although any associated infection must also be treated.

● *Nursing interventions* ●

The nursing care of surgical wounds and their complications varies. A range of common types will be considered.

Primary healing

The care of wounds healing by first intention is generally straightforward. A simple island dressing is commonly used to cover the wound at the end of the operation. Several studies have shown that the dressing can be removed after 24-48 hours and need not be replaced (Cruse & Foord, 1980; Weiss, 1983; Chrintz *et al.*, 1989). Some surgeons prefer to cover the wound with a film dressing and leave it in place

SPECIFIC ASSESSMENT FOR A PATIENT WITH SUTURED INCISION/LACERATION

Name:

Type of suture: interrupted ☐
                   continuous   ☐
                   clips   ☐
                   tape   ☐
                   none   ☐

Drains:

Type & no.:   redivac   ☐   Yes   No
               portex   ☐   Is it a
               corrugated ☐   closed system?   ☐   ☐
               other   ☐

Wound appearance   –   Location

Date	Yes	No	Yes	No	Yes	No	Yes	No	Yes	No
Clean and dry										
Localised tenderness										
Swelling of incision line										
Redness of incision line more than 1 cm										
Localised heat										
Purulent drainage										
Approximation of skin edges										
Serosanguinous drainage										

Suggested Plan:

Fig. 6.3 Suggested assessment sheet.

Based on Cuzzell, J.Z. (1986) *American Journal of Nursing*, **86** (6), 600.

until the sutures are removed. Whichever method is used, normal hygiene can be resumed and the patient may have a bath or shower.

The wound should be monitored daily for any indication of complication. Fig. 6.3 is an example of a method of recording and monitoring the progress of such a wound. Removal of sutures or other types of wound closure is usually carried out under medical supervision.

Delayed primary closure

The aim of management of these wounds is to allow free drainage of any pus. This may be achieved by loose packing of the cavity. As the wound will be sutured at about day five, the promotion of granulation is not a major aim. If ribbon gauze is used, it should be kept moist and changed regularly to prevent drying out and adherence to the wound. Alginate rope may also be used as it is very absorbent and can be removed without pain to the patient. Once the wound is sutured it should be treated as a wound healing by first intention.

Surgical cavities

Surgical cavities are generally clean wounds with a healthy bed which would be expected to heal without complication. Harding (1990) suggests that surgical cavities should be boat-shaped in order to heal rapidly without premature surface healing. Simple wound measurement is usually sufficient to monitor healing rates (see Section 4.3). The wound should also be observed for indications of infection.

Selection of a suitable dressing depends on the position of the wound and the amount of exudate. Traditionally, ribbon gauze packing, often soaked in antiseptic solutions, has been used in these wounds. Dealey (1989) and Bale (1991) have considered some of the reasons why its use is no longer the most effective way of managing cavity wounds.

Foam stents have been used for some considerable time in a variety of surgical cavities such a pilonidal sinus excision (Wood & Hughes, 1975; Marks et al., 1985). The majority of patients are capable of managing this dressing themselves, and so can be discharged from hospital without delay. A more recent study (Harding et al., 1991) found a preformed foam cavity wound dressing to be highly absorbent and easy to apply.

Alginate rope and ribbon have also been used successfully in cavity wounds. It is especially useful when there is a heavy exudate in the early stages of healing. Gupta & Foster (1991) have found alginate ribbon to be less painful to remove in comparison to traditional gauze packing. Dealey (1989) used an alginate ribbon in narrow cavity wounds and found it easy to apply and remove.

Appropriate management of surgical cavity wounds promotes rapid healing and reduces the pain and discomfort felt by the patient. Harding (1986) has described a successful healing rate of 93% to 100% in a range of cavity wounds.

Skin grafts

Skin grafts are widely used in reconstructive surgery following trauma or burns. They may also be used to repair chronic wounds such as pressure sores or leg ulcers. Skin grafting is a technique which permits the transfer of a portion of skin from one part of the body to another. There are several ways of classifying skin grafts. They can be divided into:

- Autografts   graft of patient's own skin
- Allografts   graft taken from another individual
- Xenografts   graft taken from another species

Grafts can be described according to their thickness. This depends on the amount of dermis that is included in the graft. A full-thickness graft includes the epidermis and all the dermis. A partial- or split-thickness graft includes the epidermis and some dermis. This type of graft can be cut to varying thickness depending on need. The graft can also be meshed in order to cover a larger surface area.

Other types of graft are flaps or pedicle grafts, pinch grafts and tissue cultures. Flaps may include other tissue besides skin and one part of the graft is still attached to the original site. This provides a blood supply to the graft until a new blood supply has been established. It is particularly useful in areas where the blood supply is poor and for areas of the face. An example is a gluteal rotation flap to cover the cavity of an ischial pressure sore.

Pinch grafts are small pieces of skin which have been obtained by pinching the area with forceps or lifting with a needle and slicing off with a knife. They have been used as a method of treating leg ulcers. Ryan (1987) suggests that they are only moderately successful, however, more than half the number of patients having recurrence within three months. This is because the underlying cause of ulceration remains unchanged.

Tissue culture has been developed primarily in burns units, where repeated grafting from the same donor site may be necessary for patients with large surface area burns. Tissue culture is a relatively new development. A small sample of skin about 2 cm in diameter can be used to culture epithelial sheets many times this size. One of the early studies was carried out by Gallico *et al.* (1984) on two children who had burn injuries affecting more than 95% of their body surface area. Tissue culture provided effective grafts for more than 50% of the body surface. When such extensive burns occur, autografting is very limited because of the lack of appropriate donor sites. Allografting is also used, but they do not always take. Tissue culture can reduce the the need for frequent surgery to take further grafts.

A graft may fail to 'take' for a variety of reasons. If there is an inadequate blood supply to the graft bed, the microcirculation will fail to grow into the graft and it will necrose from lack of oxygen. Equally, haematoma formation will cause separation of the graft. Infection, especially from *Pseudomonas aeruginosa* and β-haemolytic streptococcus, will also cause failure. If the graft slides out of position it will cause separation of some or all of the graft and lead to failure.

Grafts may be sutured or stapled in position or just laid in place. The graft may be left exposed or covered with a dressing to help anchor it in place. The graft must be observed carefully for any indication of infection, oedema or haematoma. It may also be necessary to immobilize the area so that the graft does not slip out of position. Tension over the graft must also be avoided as it may damage the vulnerable blood supply.

A gauze dressing is commonly used to cover the graft. If the dressing is removed, it must be done extremely carefully in order to avoid loosening the graft. Eldad & Tuchman (1987) have successfully used a hydrophilic polyurethane film as an interface between the graft and the outer dressing. The film is left in position whilst the outer dressing is changed. The researchers used it when grafting patients suffering from burn injuries and found about a 75% take, which they considered to be better than expected with these types of grafts. Vloemans (1990) used a silicone dressing material to fix 10 split-thickness skin grafts. He found 100% take in nine cases, with minor loss in one patient.

As the graft becomes vascularized it becomes approximately the same colour as the donor site. In Caucasians, the ideal colour is pink. It is more difficult to assess the vascularity of a graft in darker skins. Coull & Wylie (1990) suggest the use of a colour code along with an assessment chart to monitor the progress of skin flaps.

Once a graft has taken, it still needs to be handled very carefully as the tissues are still fragile. It should be protected against any extremes of temperature and against sunlight.

Donor sites

Ideally, donor sites are taken from a part of the body where the skin provides a good match for the recipient site. The colour, texture and hair-bearing properties of the skin have to be considered. One of the commonest areas for a donor site is the thigh, where a large area of skin can be obtained.

Donor sites are often described as being more painful than the skin graft for which the removed skin has been used. This is probably, in part, because of the large number of exposed nerve endings and, in part, because of the very traditional way that many donor sites are managed. Initially, a donor site is a raw haemorrhagic area. Pressure is needed to stop the bleeding and the wound should be checked regularly in the immediate postoperative period. Analgesia is also necessary and may be needed for several days.

Traditionally, donor sites have been dressed with paraffin gauze, covered with ordinary gauze, wrapped in wool roll or gamgee and held in place with bandages (Wilson & Taylor, 1987). The dressing is left in place for about ten days and then removed. This is often a very painful experience as the dressing has dried out and adhered to the wound. The patient may have to sit in a bath to soak the dressing off, but damage to the newly formed tissue can still occur as the dressing is pulled away. Wilson & Taylor (1987) suggest leaving the paraffin gauze *in situ* for a few days more if the gauze is adherent. Any gauze that has separated may be trimmed away. The newly epithelializing wound may be quite sore and dessicated. Lanolin or similar cream may be applied as a moisturizer – caution should be used when applying creams to check for known allergy to lanolin.

A variety of studies of caring for donor sites have demonstrated that several of the modern dressing products could be more effective than traditional methods. Studies have looked at the use of semipermeable films, hydrocolloids and alginates. Two major findings on the use of all such products are: the reduction of pain suffered by the patient and faster healing.

Film dressings were the first of the modern dressings to be used on donor sites. James & Watson (1975) evaluated the use of a film dressing and found that there was a complete absence of pain at the donor site. Patients who had previously had conventional treatment to a donor site stated their preference for the film dressing. May et al. (1984) compared the healing times of a film dressing, impregnated gauze and porcine xenograft on partial-thickness donor sites. There was a significant difference in healing rates. The mean healing times were 6.82 days for the film dressing, 9.61 days for the impregnated gauze and 12 days for the xenograft. However, one problem with film dressings is the accumulation of fluid under the film, although Golan *et al.* (1985) reported the use of a film dressing with a high water vapour permeability intended to address this problem.

The use of hydrocolloids has been studied by several researchers.

Blitz *et al.* (1985) compared a hydrocolloid dressing with saline gauze, and found a significantly faster healing time with the hydrocolloid dressing. The mean healing time was 7.2 days compared with 13.5 days with saline gauze. Pain at dressing change was also significantly less with the hydrocolloid dressing as it did not adhere to the wound. Champsaur *et al.* (1988) found similar results when comparing a hydrocolloid with paraffin gauze. They also found that the donor site was ready for re-sampling after 10 days with the hydrocolloid compared with 15 days with paraffin gauze.

Groves & Lawrence (1986) found that alginates significantly reduced the amount of blood loss from donor sites in the immediate postoperative period. Attwood (1989) compared an alginate dressing with paraffin gauze. He found that the alginate had a significantly faster healing time and provided greater comfort for the patients.

Once the donor site has healed the skin should be kept supple. The use of lanolin creams may be of assistance and should be applied two or three times a day. The patient should be advised to avoid extremes of temperature. If it is not possible to avoid exposing the site to sunlight, sunblockers should be used to cover the area. Donor sites remain susceptible to sunburn. A tubular bandage may be applied to donor sites on a lower limb to provide support and to prevent hypertrophy of the scar (Wilson & Taylor, 1987).

6.2.2 Managing complications

Dehiscence

If a surgical wound starts to break down, the potential cause(s) should be identified and rectified where possible. The wound should be carefully assessed for indications of infection. If major dehiscence, such as a burst abdomen, occurs, the wound will need resuturing. Most wounds are treated conservatively and allowed to heal by granulation and contraction. This is particularly so when infection is present, as all purulent material needs to be allowed free drainage.

The wound is often necrotic or sloughy with a heavy offensive exudate. Plate 17 shows a dehiscent wound that has broken down because of repeated surgery and poor nutrition. Parenteral feeding was commenced and the wound was managed using a calcium alginate. Plates 18 and 19 show the rapid improvement in wound appearance and reduction in wound size. Chaloner (1991) used a calcium alginate ribbon to manage a dehiscent mastectomy wound and found it provided rapid and pain-free healing. Cardy & McIntosh (1991) found calcium alginate dressing effective in managing broken down vein graft donor sites on the leg.

If there is only a partial dehiscence of the suture line with little exudate and necrosis, as shown in Plate 19 then an amorphous hydrogel is appropriate. Any small cavity can be filled with hydrogel using a syringe and filling cannula. This causes far less trauma than using traditional methods such as ribbon gauze. Once any cavity is filled with granulation tissue and there is no indication of lingering infection, foam cavity fillers may also be used.

In a few instances the exudate may be excessive and not controlled by dressings. Here it may be helpful to consult the stoma nurse, who may suggest that an appliance similar to a drainage bag be used. This has an adhesive backing which can be cut to fit over the wound, whilst protecting the surrounding skin. The front of the appliance has a hinged lid which allows access to the wound and saves frequent removal. There is usually a tap which allows drainage. The amount of exudate can be measured accurately which is important for fluid balance.

Good management of a wound following dehiscence should promote healing and permit the patient to be discharged home for care in the community.

Sinus formation

Although wide excision is the most appropriate method of managing a sinus, it is not always possible. If the sinus is very deep the opening may be fairly narrow in relation to the sinus size. Everett (1985) suggests that inserting a drainage tube into the sinus will prevent the sinus closing and allow free drainage. The tube can gradually be withdrawn as the sinus heals.

Fistulae

The management of fistulae involves care of the surrounding skin, containing and measuring the output and nutritional support. The skin can be protected by the use of ostomy pastes and protective skin wafers. Drainage bags can be applied to collect the output from the fistula. The stoma nurse may have the greatest skill in applying a suitable drainage bag over the fistula and protecting the skin.

Occasionally, it is not possible to retain a drainage bag over a fistula. In circumstances such as these, a suction tube can then be inserted by the medical staff and attached to a low pressure suction machine. There is likely to be some leakage around the tube, however. The skin should therefore be protected with protective wafer and a dressing applied to absorb the fluid.

Once the output from the fistula is contained it can be accurately measured. This enables the correct amount of fluid to be given to replace what has been lost. In hospitals where there is a nutrition team, they can also be involved in the care of these patients. When it is possible, enteral feeding should be given. If the fistula is high in the gastrointestinal tract then it will be necessary to give parenteral nutrition.

Management of fistulae requires skilled nursing care. Felice (1990), Krasner (1990) and North (1990) have provided case histories to demonstrate how fistulae can be managed. Whilst some fistulae may resolve spontaneously, others will require surgical intervention. For this latter group, nursing care can only be seen to contain the problem, not resolve it.

● *Evaluation* ●

Regular monitoring of surgical wounds is essential in order to identify any potential complications. Early intervention may prevent further problems.

6.3 TRAUMATIC WOUNDS

Traumatic injuries can range from a simple cut to a major crushing injury. Major traumatic injury is beyond the remit of this book. It requires surgical intervention and specialized nursing care. Further information about these types of wounds can be obtained from the reading list at the end of this chapter. Most nurses will be required to care for minor traumatic wounds from time to time. Their care will be considered here.

6.3.1 Minor traumatic wounds

● *Assessment* ●

Initial assessment should be to identify any life-threatening problems, such as airway obstruction, haemorrhage or shock. Vital signs should be recorded. Any of these problems should be addressed before treating the wound.

If possible, a history should be obtained of when, where and how the injury occurred. A medical history can highlight any factors which may affect healing of the wound. This information may also affect the type of treatment prescribed to manage the wound. Wounds can be divided into clean or dirty categories. Brunner & Suddarth (1989) describe clean wounds as those which occurred indoors, less than 6 hours previously; a dirty wound is one which occured outside, bleeds, and is more than 6 hours old or one which may have been sustained whilst the patient was handling soil, animals, skins or raw meat. The patient's tetanus immunity should also be acertained.

The wound should be assessed for any bleeding. Haemorrhage may be resolved by pressure or require surgical intervention. The presence of any foreign bodies should be noted and the extent and severity of the injury. Cleansing of the wound may be necessary before a full assessment can be made. Loose particles may be washed off by using a 'soapy' cleanser such as Savlon ℠. Some accident and emergency departments use cling film to cover a wound until seen by the doctor. This has the advantage of keeping the wound warm and moist and allowing easy observation.

● *Nursing intervention* ●

Medical assessment and prescription may be necessary before the wound can be dressed. Although many nurses are competent to dress minor injuries, the following guidelines should be considered:

Patients should be examined by a doctor if –

- they present at an accident and emergency department
- the nature and extent of the injury is uncertain
- there is persistent bleeding
- suturing is required
- a foreign body is present
- tetanus prophylaxis may be necessary

- the injury occurred to a hospital patient
- the nurse is uncertain of the appropriate management
- it is required by nursing policies.

Prior to dressing, the wound should be thoroughly cleaned with saline. Any loose devitalized tissue should be removed. In some instances it may be necessary to shave the area around the wound if there are hairs which may interfere with the healing process. An appropriate dressing can then be applied.

Tetanus prophylaxis will be required if the patient has not had a complete course of tetanus toxoid or if no booster dose has been given for more than five years. Depending on the cause of the wound, the doctor may also prescribe a course of antibiotics.

If the patient is not an inpatient, he and/or any carer will require information about the management of the wound. Information should also be given concerning who to contact if any complication occurs. Potential complications such as fever, swelling around the wound, excessive pain or offensive discharge should be described to the patient. Ideally, this information should also be available in written form so that the patient has it for future reference.

Traumatic injuries occur primarily to the young and the elderly. Whilst most young people will heal easily, this is not necessarily true for the older people. They may need to be admitted to hospital for further care. Wijetunge (1992) has provided a useful overview of a management plan for soft-tissue injuries.

● *Evaluation* ●

The aim of any treatment is uncomplicated healing of the wound with restoration of function and minimal scarring (Bruner & Suddarth, 1988). Evaluation of minor traumatic wounds may be carried out by those making the original assessment, or the patient may be referred to the family practitioner. The majority of these wounds will heal without complication.

6.3.2 The management of specific types of traumatic wounds

Abrasions

An abrasion is a superficial injury where the skin is rubbed or torn. It can be caused by falling on a gritty surface. It may be extremely sore. Abrasions should be cleaned carefully to ensure that there are no foreign bodies embedded in the wound. Selection of a suitable dressing depends on the extent and depth of the injury. For the majority of abrasions a simple, low-adherent dressing would be appropriate. If the abrasion is very sore, a film dressing or a thin hydrocolloid can be applied. The effect of such a dressing is to keep the nerve endings from drying out. This appears to be the factor which reduces the pain.

Lacerations

A laceration is a wound which penetrates the skin and has a torn and jagged edge.

The best way to manage these wounds is to bring the skin edges together to heal by first intention. This may be achieved by the use of sutures, adhesive strips or glue. The choice of material depends on the position of the wound, its extent and the condition of the damaged skin. Suturing is recommended around joints or on the hand where movement is involved. Glue may be particularly useful for small children as it is quicker to apply than sutures. Prior to closing the wound it should be carefully cleaned and examined for any foreign bodies.

One of the commonest positions for a laceration is the pretibial laceration (see Plate 20). If this was inflicted on a young person with healthy skin, sutures or adhesive strips would probably be used. Sutures would cause tearing in the same injury in an elderly person with fragile skin. In such circumstances, adhesive strips or glue would be more suitable. Plate 21 shows a pretibial laceration with the skin edges taped together. Healing may be promoted in an elderly person by resting and elevating the affected leg.

In some centres, when treating elderly people with lacerations, paraffin gauze and paste bandages are applied over the taped laceration to provide protection and support to the wound. Paskins et al. (1988) compared this practice with the application of a hydrocolloid dressing for people with pretibial lacerations who were aged 55 years or more. They found no difference in the healing time or cosmetic result. However, the hydrocolloid dressing was preferred by the patients because of the ease of dressing change and because they could take a bath. If healing is not achieved, a skin graft may be necessary.

If there is any risk of infection as a result of severe contamination of the wound at the time of injury, primary closure is not appropriate. Conservative treatment with antibiotics and the use of dressings such as an amorphous hydrogel is preferable. An iodine-impregnated low adherent dressing may also be used for a short period of time. Once there is no likelihood of infection the use of a hydrogel or hydrocolloid is more suitable.

Fingertip injuries

Crushing fingertip injuries are very common in children. They are mainly caused by fingers being caught in house or car doors. Buckles (1985) suggests that 14% of children below the age of thirteen years suffer from this type of injury. Cockerill & Sweet (1993) describe the procedure of trephining to remove a haematoma from the nail bed. They also suggest that an X-ray may be necessary to identify any fracture. In those circumstances, prophylactic antibiotics may be needed.

The use of adhesive tapes over the finger tip can be an effective way of holding the wound edges together. The finger can then be protected by a tubular bandage. Paraffin gauze dressings have also been used on these types of injury. Sayers & Porter (1988) compared the use of paraffin gauze with a hydrocolloid dressing on finger tip injuries in adults. They found no difference in healing times. Dressing change was easier with the hydrocolloid dressing. The patients preferred its greater conformability and reduced functional restriction. The hydrocolloid dressing was found to be cheaper to use and took less nursing time. A smaller study in children found similar results. The researchers felt that the easier dressing change with the hydrocolloid was preferable when caring for frightened children.

Dog bite

In recent years, the incidence of individuals being bitten by a dog seems to have increased. A study in the USA, Klein (1989) estimated the incidence of animal bites to be between 1 million and 3.5 million each year, resulting in more than 10 000 hospital admissions. Dog bites account for 90% of the total. Castille (1991) notes that the treatment of dog bites in an accident and emergency department peaked during August. Dog bites are a greater hazard in warm weather when fewer clothes are worn.

Castille (1991) has reviewed the management of dog bites of varying severity. The injury can range from cuts and lacerations to a crush injury with associated fracture. One particularly difficult wound to manage is a puncture wound. Here, there may be devitalized tissue in the wound, particularly with crush injuries. The wound must be considered a dirty wound. Antibiotics and tetanus toxoid may be prescribed.

Careful cleansing is essential in order to assess the extent of the injury. Saline or an antimicrobial such as povidone iodine should be used. Surgical debridement or exploration may be necessary to remove devitalized tissue, skin tags or any foreign bodies. Large cuts will need suturing. Where possible, the skin edges should be brought together and sutured or taped. Puncture wounds should be left open because of the risk of infection. All wounds should be protected. An iodine-impregnated low-adherent dressing may be suitable, unless there is a moderate to heavy exudate.

6.4 THE BURN INJURY

Burns are traumatic wounds, but because of the specialized care required, they need to be considered separately from other traumatic wounds. Generally, adults with more than 15% burns or children with more than 10% burns are treated in specialized burns units. In addition, patients with deep burns of a smaller surface area or on areas of the body such as the face may be admitted to a burns unit. Patients with less serious burns may be found in any area, although in some areas they may also be taken to specialized units. Extensive description of burn care is beyond the remit of this book; a reading list can be found at the end of the chapter.

6.4.1 Aetiology

A burn is an injury caused by excessive heat. It primarily damages the skin, causing tissue destruction and coagulation of the blood vessels of the affected area. Burns are also often surrounded by an area of erythema.

Burns can be divided into four categories:

Thermal   These are caused by flame, hot water or steam, other hot liquids, and hot surfaces. Smoke inhalation injuries may be associated with fire casualties.

Chemical   Caused by spillage of strong acids, alkalis or other corrosive substances, these burns are usually industrial injuries. Damage to vital organs can occur if the chemicals are absorbed into the blood supply.

Electrical   These burns are caused by an electrical current passing through the body. The internal damage may be considerably greater than is obvious from the skin appearance. Such burns may also be associated with thermal injury.

Radiation   Radiation burns are due to overexposure to industrial ionizing radiation or following radiotherapy treatment. (Reactions to radiotherapy are covered in more detail in Section 6.5.)

Although burn injuries are usually described as accidental, it has been suggested that some individuals are more likely to suffer from them than others. This has been summarized by Boore *et al.* (1987) who divided the predisposing factors into personal and environmental.

Personal factors include:

Age   Children under school age are the most likely sufferers, but the very old are also vulnerable.

Sex   In the under-65-years age group, more males than females have suffered burns.

Physical disability   Individuals suffering from obesity, epilepsy or neurological and cardiovascular disease resulting in some degree of physical disability are vulnerable.

Psychiatric problems   Individuals with a variety of problems such as alcohol or drug abuse, behavioural difficulties, a history of suicide attempts or self-destructive behaviour or a known psychiatric condition.

Environmental factors include:

Family stress   Major life events resulting in stress, such as moving house, social isolation, family conflicts, financial difficulties or other stressors which may be found to be present at the time of injury.

Socioeconomic factors   There is an increased risk to all family members when they live in poor, overcrowded accommodation, particularly if there is also unemployment or the wage earner has an unskilled or semiskilled job.

6.4.2 Incidence in the UK

Lawrence (1989) has suggested that about 150 000 people are taken to accident and emergency departments each year suffering from burns or scalds. Furthermore, about 10% of these people require hospital admission. In a more recent report, Lawrence (1992) suggests that 1 child in every 140 under school age will be admitted to hospital with thermal injury. Many of these will be scalds. Scalds are 40 times more common in children than adults. Lawrence (1992) also noted that 40% of injuries from scalds are related to tea making, if kettle scalds are included.

One worrying factor related to this report on the epidemiology of burns is that there is no sign of any decline in the numbers of injuries each year, particularly in the numbers of affected children. This is particularly distressing when the suffering to the individual and the family are considered. However, mortality rates have gradually declined during this century to an annual rate of about 700 persons (Lawrence & Wilkins, 1986).

6.4.3 The severity of injury

The skin is the organ of the body which usually suffers the greatest damage from a burn injury. Depending on the extent of the injury, several layers may be affected. It is common to describe the severity of a burn according to its depth and extent. Burns are divided into superficial, partial-thickness and full-thickness, according to depth.

Superficial burns Only the upper strata of the epithelium are damaged. The stratum basale is unaffected.
Partial thickness burns These burns extend beyond the epidermis into the dermis.
Full-thickness burns There is full destruction of the epidermis and dermis. The damage extends into the subcuticular layer and may involve muscle and bone.

The extent of the burn is determined by the measurement of the surface area of the affected part, excluding erythema. This is described in terms of a percentage of the whole body. Various methods of achieving this have been described. An *ad hoc*

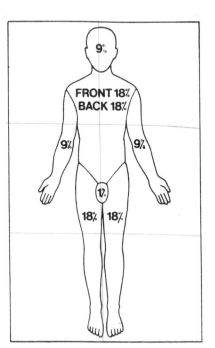

Fig. 6.4 The 'Rules of Nine'.

From: Wallace, A.B. (1951) *Lancet* i, 501.

method is to measure the area using the palm of the hand. The palmar surface of the patient is equal to 1% of the body surface area in adults and 1.5% in children. When making the initial assessment of a burn injured patient, it is most common to use the 'Rules of Nine' (Wallace, 1951). Fig. 6.4 shows how the body is divided into sections, each measuring 9% of the whole, or multiples of 9%. The percentages for

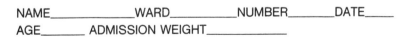

CHART FOR ESTIMATING SEVERITY OF BURN WOUND

NAME_____WARD_____NUMBER_____DATE_____
AGE_____ ADMISSION WEIGHT_____

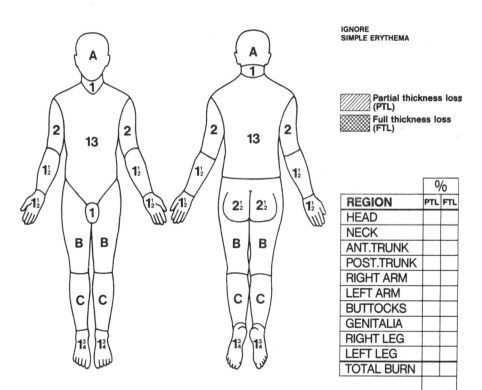

LUND AND BROWDER CHARTS

IGNORE
SIMPLE ERYTHEMA

Partial thickness loss (PTL)
Full thickness loss (FTL)

REGION	% PTL	FTL
HEAD		
NECK		
ANT.TRUNK		
POST.TRUNK		
RIGHT ARM		
LEFT ARM		
BUTTOCKS		
GENITALIA		
RIGHT LEG		
LEFT LEG		
TOTAL BURN		

RELATIVE PERCENTAGE OF BODY SURFACE AREA
AFFECTED BY GROWTH

AREA	AGE 0	1	5	10	15	ADULT
A=1/2 OF HEAD	9½	8½	6½	5½	4½	3½
B=1/2 OF ONE THIGH	2¾	3¼	4	4½	4½	4¾
C=1/2 OF ONE LEG	2½	2½	2¾	3	3¼	3½

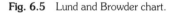

Fig. 6.5 Lund and Browder chart.

each affected area are then totalled. Thus, if one arm and the front of the trunk were affected, this would be described as 27% burns.

However, the Rule of Nines may overestimate the extent of the injury. Once the initial emergency treatment has been carried out, a reassessment of the extent of the injury is usually made. A more accurate picture can be obtained using a Lund and Browder Chart (see Fig. 6.5). Lund & Browder (1944) developed a system for assessing burn injury which not only divides the body into smaller areas, but also considers the age of the patient. Body proportions alter during childhood, so that the front of the head is 8.5% of the whole in a child of one year, but only 4.5% of the whole in a fifteen-year-old. Patient management may need to be adapted once this reassessment has been made.

6.4.4 Burn oedema

Almost immediately after injury, oedema starts to collect beneath the damaged tissue. This is typically maximal within 24 hours of the injury, but may last for up to three or four days. As plasma continues to leak into the tissues, there is a risk of hypovolaemia developing. Without treatment, hypovolaemic shock can develop and is potentially fatal. If the burn is on the face, neck or chest, the swelling from the oedema may cause obstruction of the airway. Patients with facial burns are admitted for twenty-four hours as a precaution. Treatment must ensure that the effects of burn oedema are minimized.

6.4.5 First aid treatment of burns

The British Burn Association has published recommendations for the first aid treatment of burns (Lawrence, 1987). Table 6.3 is based on these recommendations. The principle treatment is to remove the injured person from the source of heat and pour cold water over the affected area. Lawrence & Wilkins (1986)

Table 6.3 The first aid treatment of burns.

- Remove the injured person from the source of heat.
- Turn off electricity in the case of electrical burns.
- Apply copious amounts of cold water to the affected area.
- Do NOT try to remove clothing if the burns are extensive.
- Put wet compress on any exposed areas.
- Wrap cling film around wet compress to hold in place.
- Seek qualified help quickly – especially if the burn is extensive.
- If no tap water, use bottled/mineral water or milk.
- Do not use solutions such as bleach, butter or oil.

Based on Lawrence (1987).

demonstrated that the subcutaneous temperature continues to rise after the burn injury occurs. Thus, if a burn injury at 100°C lasts for 10 seconds, the affected tissue will take 3 minutes to return to normal body temperature. Application of cold water within 10 seconds of the injury can reduce the 'burn time' to 30 seconds. Lawrence calls upon on all healthcare workers, emergency service personnel and first aiders to publicize this treatment.

6.4.6 The management of burn injuries

When considering the management of burns, the extent of the injury must be defined as the treatment varies drastically between major and minor burns. Minor burns may be treated in the outpatient department, but anyone with major burns must be admitted to hospital. Lawrence (1989) has listed the criteria for hospital admission. These are:

1. Burns greater than 5% of total body area
2. Full-thickness burns greater than 10 × 10 cm
3. Deep burns over joints or flexor surfaces
4. Burns of the face
5. History of smoke inhalation or noxious vapour
6. Electrical burns
7. Chemical burns
8. Any uncertainty in relation to the above or the cause.

Major burns

The early management of major burns has been described in detail by Settle (1986). He suggests an action plan for the initial treatment of burns:

- *Check airway*   Endotracheal intubation may be needed if there are deep burns to face, neck or mouth or any indication of respiratory distress.
- *History of cause of injury*   Obtain this from patient, relative or ambulance crew. This may provide information indicating potential complications such as smoke inhalation.
- *General examination*   Identify any other obvious injury or illness and extent of burns using Rules of Nine.
- *Establish an intravenous infusion*   Essential for all burns greater than 15% of total body surface in adults and 10% in children. Blood samples may be taken at the same time.
- *Analgesia*   This may be inhalational analgesia or systemic, depending on the condition of the patient.
- *Catheterize*   If the burns are 25% or more of body total, urinary output will need to be maintained to check for inadequate rehydration as well as renal function.
- *Reassess extent of injury*   Use a Lund and Browder Chart. If there are circumferential burns on any part of the body, it may be necessary to perform escharotomy. As burn oedema forms the burned skin is unable to stretch and

thus it has a tourniquet effect. An escharotomy is a deep longitudinal incision which releases the tension.

Management of major burns is best carried out in a burns unit. If the injury occurs some considerable distance from a specialised unit, the patient may be taken first to a nearby accident and emergency department. Once the patient's condition has been stabilized by the above measures, urgent transfer can take place.

Minor burns

Managing minor burns requires assessment of both the patient and the wound as in any other type of wound. Assessment of the patient has been discussed in Chapter 3 and wound assessment in Chapter 4. Specific aspects of care can also be identified.

● *Patient assessment* ●

Maintaining a safe environment   Discover the cause of the injury. Non-accidental injury must be considered if the history seems inconsistent with the burn appearance. The risk of infection is always present in the burn-injured patient.
Communication   It is important to provide reassurance and explanation to the patient and the family. Analgesia may be required for pain.
Eating and drinking   Nutritional status should be identified. Advice on nutrition may be necessary as there will be increased nutritional demands on the body.
Mobilization   The burn injury may affect mobility. Simple exercises may be necessary.
Expressing sexuality   A burn injury can be extremely disfiguring. Body image may be profoundly altered causing distress and loss of self-esteem.
Sleeping   Pain or anxiety may affect sleep patterns.
Psychological care   Many patients will be very frightened. Specific fears should be identified and addressed. They may be fears of disfigurement or disability. Some may fear loss of loved ones as a result of the scarring.

● *Wound assessment* ●

Initial assessment of a burn injury includes the extent and depth of the burn. The use of a Lund and Browder Chart has already been described. Most burns are surrounded by an area of erythema which should not be included when calculating the burn area. Identifying the depth of a burn may not be easy. A burn injury may have varying depths. However, these guidelines may be followed:

Superficial burns

The skin looks red and dry, possibly with some oedema.

Assessment	Rationale
Pin-prick test	Pain indicates undamaged nerve endings.
Light pressure which is then released	Blanching followed by refilling of capillaries indicates undamaged blood supply.

Partial-thickness burns

In shallower partial thickness burns, the epithelium forming the shafts of the hair follicles are still intact. However, the capillary network is damaged, releasing a serous exudate which forms blisters. Beneath the blister, the wound surface appears wet, swollen and pink. Nerve endings may be exposed and the patient may experience acute pain. Deep partial thickness burns are firmer. As more blood vessels have been destroyed, there is less exudate and blistering. The colour may vary from a waxy white to a dark red.

Assessment	Rationale
Pin-prick test	Extreme pain indicates shallow partial-thickness burn; diminished sensation indicates damaged nerve endings and a deep dermal burn.
Light pressure which is then released	Indicates the degree of damage to the capillaries, the deeper the burn, the slower the refill.
The degree of blistering and exudate	The shallower the burn, the more exudate and blisters.

Full-thickness burns

The skin often looks quite leathery and dry. The colour can be black, dark brown, tan, red or white.

Assessment	Rationale
Pin-prick test	No sensation as nerve endings are destroyed.
Burn feels hard and dry	Due to coagulation of fluid in tissues.

A burn injury differs from other types of wounds in several important respects (Bayley, 1990). There are frequently large areas of devitalized tissue. The wound may have a large surface area and take some time to heal. As a result, the burn wound is rapidly colonized by bacteria. There is considerable risk of infection in major burns, but it is much less likely in minor burns. Lawrence (1989) quotes an incidence of about 1%, but this may vary between centres. Nonetheless, the wound should be observed carefully for signs of infection.

Wound management

The main goals in the management of burns are to:

- Debride burn eschar, if present
- Promote rapid healing
- Prevent/detect infection

Debridement of burn eschar can be achieved by surgical debridement or by using a dressing which will promote the autolytic processes of the body. Selection of the method will depend on the burn appearance and possibly the age of the patient. For example, surgical debridement would certainly be inappropriate in a frightened child who resisted all attempts to be held still.

The product which has been used most widely on burns is silver sulphadiazine. It is the dressing of choice for major burns until grafting can take place. Silver sulphadiazine has an antimicrobial effect and is effective against Gram-negative and *Candida* sp. It thus has the advantage of helping to prevent infection. However, high standards of asepsis are still required at dressing change.

In minor burns, other types of wound management products are also used. Small partial-thickness burns have traditionally been treated with an antiseptic-impregnated tulle or paraffin gauze dressings covered with gauze and a bandage. Although healing will occur with this regime, there are several disadvantages. The dressings are bulky and hinder washing around the affected area. They may also be painful to remove, although it may not be necessary to remove the wound contact layer until the wound is healed and it separates spontaneously.

Studies of some of the more modern products indicate that they may also have a role to play. The use of semipermeable films was studied by Neale *et al*. (1981) who found a faster healing rate than with conventional paraffin gauze. Conkle (1981) found a considerable reduction in burn pain when using a film dressing. The major disadvantage with most of the semipermeable films, however, is their lack of absorptive capacity. Smith & Rennie (1991) described the use of a highly vapour permeable film which reduced fluid build up in most of the burns so treated.

Hydrocolloids may be used and can absorb exudate. Hermans & Hermans (1986) used a hydrocolloid dressing on partial-thickness burns and found that there was a good healing rate with minimal scarring. The dressing was comfortable to wear and reduced wound pain. Phipps & Lawrence (1988) compared a hydro-colloid dressing with medicated tulle dressings. The healing rates were comparable and the hydrocolloid was found to be easy to apply.

Other dressings that can be used on minor burns include flat foam dressings and hydrogels. The foam dressings are comfortable and can be held in place with tape or a tubular net. Hydrogels can give a cooling sensation when applied which may be comforting to the patient.

Burns of the hands are best treated with silver sulphadiazine. Once the cream is applied the hand should be covered by a plastic bag. This will allow free movement and help to prevent contractures. There are, however, several disadvantages with the use of plastic bags. They cause considerable maceration of the whole hand as large quantities of exudate accumulate in the bag. The bag becomes heavy and pulls the wrist into flexion. Once full of fluid, the bag tends to leak or tear, necessitating dressing change. Terrill *et al*. (1991) compared the use of Gore-Tex ™ bags with plastic bags. Gore-Tex ™ has the property of water vapour permeability. Although there was no difference in healing times, there was a considerable reduction in skin maceration and accumulation of exudate when using Gore-Tex ™. Improved hand function was also noted. Witchell & Crossman (1991) compared the use of these bags over silver sulphadiazine with paraffin gauze for children with burns of the hands. They found that use of Gore-Tex ™ bags increased child activity and reduced the length of time of dressing change. More significantly, there were considerably

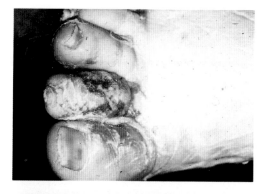

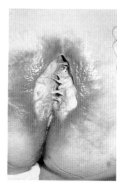

Plate 1 (far left) A necrotic wound.

Plate 2 (left) An infected wound.

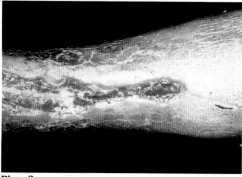

Plate 3

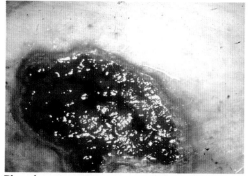

Plate 4

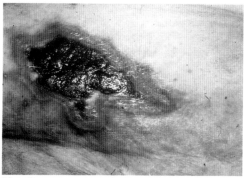

Plate 5

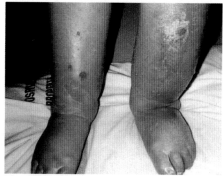

Plate 6

Plate 3 A sloughy wound.

Plate 4 A granulating wound.

Plate 5 An epithelializing wound.

Plate 6 Oedematous legs with fragile skin and ulcers.

Plate 7 The same – one week later.

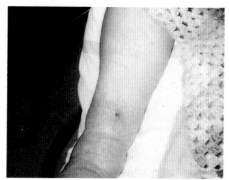

Plate 7

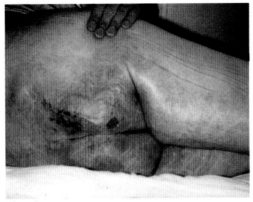

Plate 8

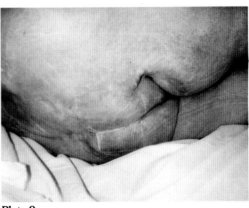

Plate 9

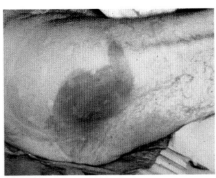

Plate 10

Plate 8 A patient with allergies to several dressings.

Plate 9 The same after application of protective skin wipe.

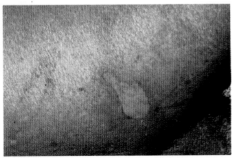

Plate 11

Plate 10–13 Pressure sore grades.

Plate 10 Stage I: non blanchable erythema of intact skin.

Plate 11 Stage II: partial-thickness skin loss involving epidermis and/or dermis.

Plate 12 Stage III: full-thickness wound involving epidermis, dermis and subcuticular layer.

Plate 13 Stage IV: Extensive destruction involving other tissues such as muscle, tendon and bone.

Plate 12

Plate 13

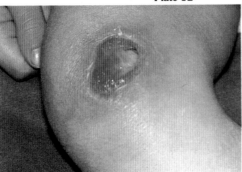

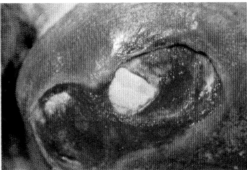

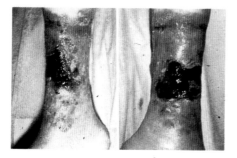

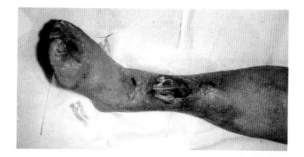

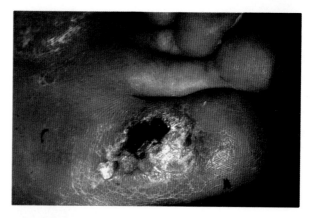

Plate 14 (above, left) A typical venous ulcer.

Plate 15 (above, right) An arterial ulcer.

Plate 16 (right) A neuropathic ulcer.

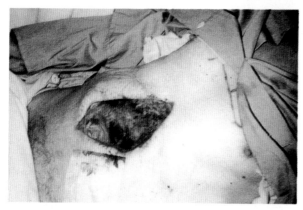

Plate 17 The dehiscence of an abdominal wound.

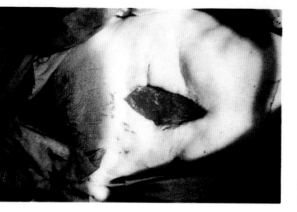

Plate 18 The wound can now be managed in the community.

Plate 19 Minor breakdown in a suture line.

Plate 20 A pretibial laceration.

Plate 21 Taping a pretibial laceration.

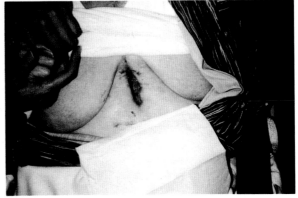

Plate 19

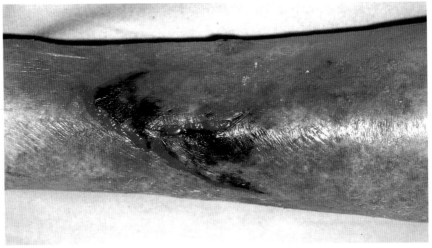

Plate 20

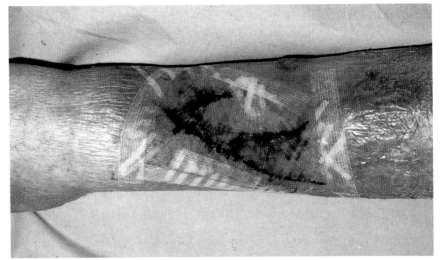

Plate 21

fewer unscheduled visits to the accident and emergency department because of problems with the dressing. This type of bag may be more widely available in the future.

● *Evaluation* ●

Evaluation of the burns wound involves both monitoring of the wound as it progresses towards healing and of the healed wound. Once the wound is healed, special care needs to be taken of the newly formed epithelia. Bayley (1990) suggests cleansing with a mild soap and then applying water-based cream several times a day. The patient should be warned to avoid any possibility of sun burn.

Potential problems which can develop are contractures and hypertrophic scarring. Myofibroblasts contract and shorten the wound, causing the collagen fibres to become coiled. The scar develops a hard, red, raised appearance. If the burn injury is over a joint, as the myofibroblasts contract it causes flexion of the joint. Unless measures are taken to splint the joint, it will become contracted. A programme of exercise and splinting to counteract this will be established by the physiotherapist as appropriate. Hypertrophic scarring is usually managed by the wearing of pressure garments. In effect, they squash it flat. They are usually custom-made and have to be worn for about a year. An alternative treatment, using a silicone gel sheet, has been considered by Ahn *et al.* (1989). They found it to be an acceptable alternative to pressure garments over small areas. Further research by Carney *et al.* (1993) of 42 patients found that the gel needed to be worn for a minimum of 12 hours a day. This study lasted for two months during which time definite improvements were found. However, further research is needed to provide a clearer indication of the length of time the gel should be used on a scar.

A few patients will develop permanent pigmentation changes. This is possibly because of damage to the melanocytes in the basal layer of the epidermis. It can present as either apigmentation or hyperpigmentation. It is not possible to predict when it will occur.

The management of burns is complex and requires specialized knowledge. Suggestions for further reading are listed at the end of the chapter.

6.5 RADIATION REACTIONS

A radiation reaction is the reaction of the skin to the effects of radiotherapy and is limited to the treatment field or its exit point. Strictly speaking, a radiation reaction is not a wound. However, the skin reaction is akin to a superficial burn and has the potential for ulceration. There is insufficient research into the management of what can be a very painful problem.

6.5.1 Aetiology

Ionizing radiation or radiotherapy is the mainstay of cancer treatment. Treatment is usually given in a series of doses, ranging from daily to weekly, although a small number of patients will receive just one dose. A course of treatment may last up to eight weeks. Radiation reactions are most likely to occur when the treatment field is close to the body surface, such as the head or neck, or if it includes axillae, under breasts, perineum or groin. The reaction is dose-dependent – that is, the more frequent the treatment or the higher the dose, the more likely the reaction. Some individuals are more likely to have reaction than others. In particular, blonds are much more vulnerable than those with a darker skin, although those with a dark skin may also have severe reactions. A reaction may occur during a course of treatment or after it is completed. Within six weeks of completion of treatment, all but the most severe reactions have disappeared.

6.5.2 The classification of radiation reactions

Yasko (1982) classified radiation reactions as follows:

Stage I: Inflammation
Erythema of the area which can vary from pink to bright red. There may be slight oedema.
Stage II: Desquamation (dry)
Erythema plus a dry appearance to the skin can be seen, due to damage to the sebaceous glands in the treatment field. There may be skin irritation or a slight burning sensation.
Stage III: Desquamation (wet)
At this stage, erythema, oedema and blistering can be seen. In the event of such a severe reaction, radiotherapy is usually stopped until it has resolved.
Stage IV: Epilation, fibrosis and atrophy
High doses of radiation can cause permanent hair loss to the site and damage to the sebaceous and/or sweat glands. In turn, this may result in later side-effects such as damage to the lymphatic drainage or telangiectasis.

A small study of women being treated for breast cancer found that they all had skin reactions of varying degrees (Lawton & Twoomey, 1991). The worst reactions occurred within three weeks of completing treatment and lasted for several weeks. The commonest reaction was tenderness and itching. This occurred in 65% of the sample. Other reactions included tightness of skin, erythema and moist desquamation, the latter occurring in 45% of the women.

6.5.3 Management of the skin

There is considerable confusion concerning how the skin within the treatment field should be managed whilst radiotherapy is in progress. A survey by Thomas (1992) found that there is no uniformity of opinion among radiotherapy centres. Some suggest that the skin should not be washed at all during the course of treatment. This is highly unacceptable to patients. Others suggest that the area may be washed with water only and patted dry, taking care not to remove the special markings indicating the treatment field. Another area of disagreement is the use of powders. Some would say that no talcum powder should be used whilst others would suggest starch powder might be used. Starch powder, unlike other talcum powders, does not contain metal particles which would scatter the rays. A common example of starch powder is baby powder. It should be noted that all of these directions are based on anecdotal evidence. Thomas calls for a definitive study to determine the most appropriate skin care.

There certainly seems to have been little research interest in this area. However, one study is available for reference, that of Lawton & Twoomey (1991). They suggest that there seems to be no benefit in not allowing the patient to wash the treatment area, as long as unperfumed soaps are used and the skin patted dry.

There has also been little research into the management of radiation reactions. However, they can be classed as a minor burn and basic principles of wound care can provide some guidelines.

Stage I   Treat as sunburn and apply simple emollients which do not contain metals, such as zinc.

Stage II   A simple emollient cream may be used. Thomas (1992) found that a wide range of creams are in use, the most popular being hydrocortisone cream, but that little research has been undertaken to support any particular selection. The study by Lawton & Twoomey (1991) found the use of a hydrocortisone cream conferred no added benefit. They suggest that Calendula cream may have a greater effect.

Stage III   A range of modern wound management products can be used. Shell (1984) found film dressings more effective than paraffin gauze. Margolin *et al.* (1990) found that using a hydrocolloid dressing considerably reduced pain as well as promoting healing. Pickering & Warland (1992) compared a sheet hydrogel with gentian violet and exposure to air. They found that the hydrogel reduced discomfort and decreased healing time. Lober & Panduro (1993) used a silicone dressing on 13 patients with moist desquamation all of whom found it provided relief from discomfort. It would seem that the principles of modern wound management can be applied effectively to areas of wet desquamation.

Stage IV   No specific dressings are required. Lymphoedema may develop at a later date and require management. (See Section 5.4).

6.5.4 Care of the patient

The most important aspect of care of any patient undergoing radiotherapy must be communication. Frith (1991) has reviewed the literature regarding information related to radiotherapy and concluded that patients often receive little or no information prior to treatment. This results in many unmet needs. She describes the type of information that patients need, such as what side-effects to expect and how they can be managed. Written information can be used to reinforce verbal explanations. This provides the patient with a permanent record which can be shared with others.

6.5.5 Future developments

There is obviously a need for further research into this aspect of patient care. Jackson (1993) has reported on the background to a study which is yet to be completed. Patients with malignant disease have been shown to be deficient of essential fatty acids (EFAs). The situation is exacerbated in those receiving radiotherapy. These patients are more likely to have radiation reactions. Anecdotal evidence suggested to the researchers that the use of oral evening primrose oil which contains an EFA may be beneficial. The study will compare the effect of giving evening primrose oil with a placebo to women undergoing radiotherapy for breast cancer. The side effects of the radiation treatment will be carefully monitored. This study may result in the reduction of a distressing problem.

FURTHER READING

Beaver, B.M. (1990) Trauma. *Nursing Clinics of North America* **25**, 1.
Cason, J.S. (1981) *Treatment of Burns.* Chapman and Hall, London.
Muir, I.F.K., Barclay, T.L. & Settle, J.A.D. (1987) *Burns and their Treatment* (3rd edn). Butterworth, Oxford.
Westaby, S. (1985) *Wound Care.* William Heinemann Medical Books Ltd., London.

REFERENCES

Ahn, S.T., Monafo, W.W. & Mustoe, T.A. (1989) Topical silicone gel: a new treatment for hypertrophic scars. *Surgery* **106**: 4, 781–7.
Attwood, A. (1989) Calcium alginate dressing accelerates split skin graft donor site healing. *British Journal of Plastic Surgery* **42**, 373–9.
Bale, S. (1991) A holistic approach and the ideal dressing: cavity wound management in the 1990s. *Professional Nurse* **6**: 6, 316–23.
Bayley, E.W. (1990) Wound healing in the patient with burns. *Nursing Clinics of North America* **25**: 1, 205–22.
Bell, F.G. & Fenton, P.A. (1993) Early hospital discharge and cross infection. *Lancet* **342**: 8863, 120.
Bibby, B.A., Collins, B.J. & Ayliffe, G.A.J. (1986) A mathematical model for assessing the risk of postoperative wound infection. *Journal of Hospital Infection* **8**, 31–9.
Blitz, H., Kiessling, M. & Kreysel, H.A. (1985) Comparison of hydrocolloid dressing and saline gauze in the treatment of skin graft donor sites. In Ryan, T.J. (ed) *An Environment for Healing: The Role of Occlusion.* Royal Society of Medicine, London.
Boore, J., Champion, R. & Ferguson, M.C. (1987) *Nursing the Physically Ill Adult.* Churchill Livingstone, Edinburgh.
Brunner, L.S. & Suddarth, D.S. (1988) *Textbook of Medical-Surgical Nursing.* J.B. Lippincott Company, Philadelphia.
Brunner, L.S. & Suddarth, D.S. (1989) *The Lippincott Manual of Medical-Surgical Nursing.* Harper & Row, London.
Buckles, E. (1985) Wound care in accident and emergency. *Nursing* **2**: 42, suppl. 3–5.
Bucknall, T.E., Cox, P.J. & Ellis, H. (1982) Burst abdomen and incisional hernia: a prospective study of 1129 laparotomies. *British Medical Journal* **284**, 931–33.

Cardy, M.A. & McIntosh, A. (1991) *Management of wound dehiscence using a calcium alginate dressing.* 4th Annual Symposium on Advanced Wound Care, San Francisco.

Carney, S.A., Cason, C.G. & Gowar, J.P. (1993) Treating hypertrophic scars with silicone gel. *Journal of Wound Care* **2**: 4, 197–98.

Castille, K. (1991) Once bitten... *Nursing Times* **87**: 39, 26–28.

Chaloner, D. (1991) Treating a cavity wound. *Nursing Times* **87**: 13, 67–69.

Champsaur, A., Amadou, R., Nefzi, A. & Marichy, J. (1988) Use of Duoderm on donor sites after skin grafting. A comparative study with tulle-gras. In Ryan, T.J. (ed) *Beyond Occlusion: Wound Care Proceedings.* Royal Society of Medicine, London.

Chrintz, H., Vibits, H., Cordtz, T.O. *et al.* (1989) Need for surgical wound dressing. *British Journal of Surgery* **76**, 204–5.

Cockerill, J. & Sweet, A. (1993) Nursing management of common accident wounds. *British Journal of Nursing* **2**: 11, 578–82.

Conkle, W.J. (1981) Opsite dressing: a new approach to burn care. *Emergency Nursing* **7**: 4, 148–52.

Coull, A. & Wylie, K. (1990) Regular monitoring: the way to ensure flap healing. *Professional Nurse* **6**: 1, 18–21.

Cruse, P.J.E. & Foord, R.(1973) A five-year prospective study of 23,649 surgical wounds. *Archives of Surgery* **107**, 206–10.

Cruse, P.J.E. & Foord, R. (1980) The epidemiology of wound infection, a ten-year prospective study of 62,939 wounds. *Surgical Clinics of North America* **60**: 1, 27–40.

Dealey, C. (1989) Management of cavity wounds. *Nursing* **3**: 39, 25–27.

Dealey, C. (1991) Managing surgical wounds. *Nursing* **4**: 43, 29–32.

Eldad, A. & Tuchman, I. (1987) *The use of Omiderm as an interface for skin grafting.* International Congress of Burn Injuries, Geneva.

Everett, W.G. (1985) Wound sinus or fistula? In Westaby, S. (ed) *Wound Care.* William Heinemann Medical Books Ltd, London.

Felice, M.M. (1990) Draining wound management: techniques for skin preservation. In Krasner, D. (ed) *Chronic Wound Care: A Clinical Source Book for Healthcare Professionals.* Health Management Publications Inc., King of Prussia, Pennsylvania.

Frith, B. (1991) Giving information to radiotherapy patients. *Nursing Standard* **5**: 34, 33–35.

Gallico, G.G., O'Connor, N.E., Compton, C.C., Kehinde, O. & Green, H. (1984) Permanent cover of large burn wounds with autologous cultured human epithelium. *New England Journal of Medicine* **311**, 448–51.

Golan, J., Eldad, A., Rudensky, B., Tuchman, Y., Sterenberg, N., Ben-Hur, N., Behar, D. & Juszynski, M. (1985) A new temporary synthetic skin. *Burns* **11**, 274–80.

Groves, A.R. & Lawrence, J.C. (1986) Alginate dressing as a donor site haemostat. *Annals of the Royal College of Surgeons of England* **68**, 27–28.

Gupta, R., Foster, M.E. & Miller, E. (1991) Calcium alignate in the management of acute surgical wounds and abscesses. *Journal of Tissue Viability* **1**: 4, 115–16.

Harding, K.G. (1986) Clinical experience of Silastic Foam dressing. In Turner, T.D., Schmidt, R.J. & Harding, K.G. (eds) *Advances in Wound Management.* John Wiley & Sons, Chichester.

Harding, K.G., Butterworth, R., Bale, S. & Hughes, L.E. (1991) *The results of a clinical study of the efficacy and benefits of using a unique cavity wound dressing for cavity wounds.* 4th Symposium on Advanced Wound Care, San Francisco, April.

Hermans, M.H.E. & Hermans, R.P. (1986) Duoderm, an alternative dressing for small burns. *Burns* **12**: 3, 214–19.

Jackson, B. (1993) Can oral fatty acid supplements moderate radiation reactions? *Wound Management* **4**: 2, suppl. 7.

James, J.H. & Watson, A.C.H. (1975) The use of Opsite on skin graft donor sites. *British Journal of Plastic Surgery* **28**, 107–110.

Klein, J.D. (1989) Animal bite infections. *Delaware Medical Journal* **61**: 1, 17–20.

Krasner, D. (1990) Managing draining wounds: fistulae, leaking tubes and drains. In Krasner, D. (ed) *Chronic Wound Care: A Clinical Source Book for Healthcare Professionals.* Health Management Publications Inc., King of Prussia, Pennsylvania.

Lawrence, J.C. (1987) British Burn Association recommended first aid for burns and scalds. *Burns* **13**: 2, 153.

Lawrence, J.C. (1989) Treating minor burns. *Nursing Times* **85**: 26, 69–73.

Lawrence, J.C. (1992) The epidemiology of burns. In Harding, K.G., Leaper, D.L. & Turner, T.D. (eds) *Proceedings of the 1st European Conference on Advances in Wound Management.* Macmillan Magazines Ltd., London.

Lawrence, J.C. & Wilkins, M.D. (1986) The epidemiology of burns. In Lawrence, J.C. (ed.) *Burncare.* Smith and Nephew Medical Ltd., Hull.

Lawton, J. & Twoomey, M. (1991) Skin reactions to radiotherapy. *Nursing Standard* **6**: 10, 53–54.

Leigh, D.A. (1981) An eight-year study of postoperative wound infection in two district general hospitals. *Journal of Hospital Infection* **2**, 207–17.

Lober, J. & Panduro, J. (1993) Mepitel in the treatment of moist desquamation caused by radiotherapy. In Harding, K.G., Cherry, G., Dealey, C. & Turner, T.D. (eds) *Proceedings of the 2nd European Conference on Advances in Wound Management.* Macmillan Magazines Ltd., London.

Lund, C.C. & Browder, N.C. (1944) Estimations of areas of burns. *Surgery, Gynaecology and Obstetrics* **79**, 352.

Margolin, S.G., Breneman, J.C., Denman, D.L., LaChapelle, P., Weckbach, L. & Aron, B.S. (1990) Management of radiation-induced moist skin desquamation using hydrocolliod dressing. *Cancer Nursing* **13**: 2, 71–80.

Marks, J., Harding, K.G., Hughes, L.E. & Ribeiro, C.D. (1985) Pilonidal sinus excision healing by open granulation. *British Journal of Surgery* **72**, 637–40.

May, S.R., Karandy, E.J., Burgos, S.M., *et al.* (1984) Moist wound healing of autograft skin donor sites. *The Bulletin and Clinical Review of Burn Injuries* **1**: 2, 36.

Mishriki, S.F., Law, D.J.W. & Jeffery, P.T. (1990) Factors affecting the incidence of postoperative wound infection. *Journal of Hospital Infection* **16**, 223–30.

Neale, D.E., Whalley, P.C., Flowers, M.W. & Wilson, D.H. (1981) The effects of an adherent polyurethane film and conventional absorbent dressing in patients with small partial thickness burns. *British Journal of Clinical Practice* **35**: 7/8, 254–57.

North, A.P. (1990) Management of an enterovaginal fistula. In Krasner, D. (ed) *Chronic Wound Care: a Source Book for Healthcare Professionals.* Health Management Publications Inc., King of Prussia, Pennsylvania.

Paskins, J.R., Crosby, A.C., Ferguson, D.G. & Hockey, M. (1988) A multicentre prospective trial of Granuflex dressings vs paste bandages in the treatment of pretibial lacerations. In Ryan, T.J. (ed) *Beyond Occlusion: Wound Care Proceedings.* Royal Society of Medicine, London.

Perkins, P. (1992) Wound dehiscence: causes and care. *Nursing Standard* **6**: 34, suppl. 12–14.

Phipps, A.R. & Lawrence, J.C. (1988) Comparison of hydrocolloid dressings and medicated tulle gras in the treatment of out-patient burns. In Ryan, T.J. (ed) *Beyond Occlusion: Wound Care Proceedings.* Royal Society of Medicine, London.

Pickering, D.G. & Warland, S. (1992) The management of desquamative radiation skin reactions. *Dressing Times* **5**: 1, 1–2.

Poole, G.V. (1985) Mechanical factors in abdominal wound closure. *Surgery* **97**, 631–40.

Richold, J.C. (1992) Review of post-operative surgical wound infection in a district general hospital. In Harding, K.G., Leaper, D.L. & Turner, T.D. (ed) *Proceedings of the 1st European Conference on Advances in Wound Management.* Macmillan Magazines Ltd., London.

Ryan, T.J. (1987) *The Management of Leg Ulcers.* Oxford University Press, Oxford.

Sayers, R. & Porter, K.M. (1988) Comparison of duoderm and medicated tull-gras in the treatment of finger-tip injuries. In Ryan, T.J. (ed) *Beyond Occlusion: Wound Care Proceedings.* Royal Society of Medicine, London.

Settle, J.A.D. (1986) *Burns – The First Five Days.* Smith & Nephew Pharmaceuticals Ltd, Hull.

Shell, J. (1984) Comparison of moisture vapour permeable dressings to conventional dressings for management of radiation skin reactions. Oncology Nursing Society Conference, Toronto, Canada.

Smith, K. & Rennie, M.J. (1991) Management of burn injuries: a rationale for the use of temporary synthetic skin substitutes. *Professional Nurse* **6**: 10, 571–4.

Taylor, D.E.M., Whamond, J.S. & Penhallow, J.E. (1987) Effects of haemorrhage on wound strength and fibroblast function. *British Journal of Surgery* **74**, 316–19.

Terrill, P.J., Kedwards, S.M. & Lawrence, J.C. (1991) The use of Gore-Tex bags for hand burns. *Burns* **17**: 2, 161–5.

Thomas, S. (1992) Current practices in the management of fungating lesions and radiation-damaged skin. The Surgical Materials Testing Laboratory, Bridgend.

Torrance, C. (1993) Introduction to surgical drainage. *Surgical Nurse* **6**: 2, 19–23.

Vloemans, A.F.P.M. (1990) *The fixation of split-thickness skin grafts by Mepitel. An inventory of ten patients.* Data on file. Molnlycke Ltd., Dunstable.

Wallace, A.B. (1951) The exposure treatment of burns. *Lancet* **i**, 501–4.

Weiss, Y. (1983) Simplified management of operative wounds by early exposure. *International Surgery* **68**, 237–40.

Westaby, S. (1985) Wound closure and drainage. In Westaby, S. (ed) *Wound Care.* William Heinemann Medical Books Ltd, London.

Wijetunge, D. (1992) An A & E approach. *Nursing Times* **88**: 46, 70–76.

Wilson, A.P.R., Weavill, C., Burridge, J. & Kelsey, M.C. (1990) The use of the wound scoring method 'ASEPSIS' in postoperative wound surveillance. *Journal of Hospital Infection* **16**, 297–309.

Wilson, G.R. & Taylor, H.E. (1987) *Blueprint for the Nursing Care of the Skin Graft Donor Site.* Squibb Surgicare Ltd, Middlesex.

Witchell, M. & Crossman, C. (1991) Dressing burns in children. *Nursing Times* **87**: 36, 63–66.

Wood, R.A.B. & Hughes, L.E. (1975) Silicone foam sponge for pilonidal sinus: a new technique for managing open granulating wounds. *British Medical Journal* **3**, 131–3.

Yasko, J.M. (1982) Care of the patient receiving radiation therapy. *Nursing Clinics of North America* **17**: 4, 631–48.

Chapter 7
Three Case Studies

7.1 INTRODUCTION

There is often discussion about the gap between theory and practice. This chapter aims to fill this gap, and describes a series of case studies to demonstrate how the basic principles of wound care might be applied. They have been outlined with simple documentation and assessment forms provide a useful framework to follow.

NB: Examples of particular wound management products are given in these case studies. This should not be seen as any particular endorsement of these products.

7.2 MANAGING AN INFECTED SURGICAL INCISION

7.2.1 Background information

Mrs Cynthia Smith has had a cholecystectomy operation for gall stones. She is 45 years old, married with two teenage children. Mrs Smith is overweight, but has lost 13 kg prior to admission. The operation and immediate postoperative period were uneventful. On the third day after surgery Mrs Smith complained of feeling unwell and of having excessive pain along the suture line.

● *Patient assessment* ●

ASSESSMENT FORM FOR PATIENTS WITH OPEN WOUNDS/MAJOR SURGERY

Name: Mrs Cynthia SMITH　　　　　**Hospital No.:** 34567

Ward: 2　　　　　　　　　　　　　　**Consultant:** Mr Wright

Age: 45 yrs　　　　**Sex:** F　　　**Waterlow Score:** 8

Date of Assessment: 9 September

5 September Cholecystectomy

1. **Maintaining a Safe Environment**　　　　　　　　　　Yes　　No

   Infection

   a) Is infection present elsewhere (ie not the wound)?　☐　☑
   b) If yes to (a), is this being treated?　　　　　　　☐　☐

2. **Communicating**

   a) Are there any communication problems?　　　☐　☑
   b) If yes to (a), please specify.
   c) Does patient appear anxious?　　　　　　　☐　☑
   d) HAD score =

3. **Breathing**

   a) Has the patient known cardiovascular disease?　☐　☑
   b) Is peripheral vascular disease present?　　　　☐　☑
   c) Is oedema present?　　　　　　　　　　　　☐　☑
   d) Is there discoloration of the legs?　　　　　☐　☑
   e) Is the patient anaemic?　　　Don't know　☐　☐　☑
   f) If yes to (e), is this being treated?　　　　☐　☑

4. **Eating and Drinking**

   Nutritional Status

   a) Is the patient eating a well balanced diet?　☑　☐
      Comments:
   b) Are there signs of i) obesity?　　　　　　　　☑　☐
      　　　　　　　　ii) emaciation?　　　　　　☐　☑
      　　　　　　　iii) muscle wasting?　　　　　☐　☑
   c) Is weight within 'normal' limits?　　　　　　☐　☑
   d) Has patient lost weight recently?　　　　　　☑　☐
      Comments: 1000 kcal diet, lost 13kg prior to surgery
   e) Are plasma proteins low?　　　Don't know　☐　☐　☑
      Other comments:

   Underlying Disease

   a) Is the patient a diabetic?　　　　　　　　　☐　☑
   b) If yes to (a), is it stable at present?　　　☐　☐

   Smoking

   a) Does the patient smoke?　　　　　　　　　　☐　☑
   b) If yes to (a), is it - 0 - 20/day
      　　　　　　　　　　20 - 40/day
      　　　　　　　　　　40 - 60/day
      　　　　　　　　　　60 + /day

- 2 -

                                                              Yes   No

5. **Eliminating**

   a) Is the patient incontinent of i) urine?   ☐   ☑
                                    ii) faeces?   ☐   ☑
   b) If yes to (a), can the problem be improved? ☐   ☐
      Comments:
   c) Has the patient uraemia?   ☐   ☐
   d) Is the blood urea above 7mmol/l?   ☐   ☐
                            Don't know   ☐

6. **Mobilising**

   a) Is the patient fully mobile?   ☐   ☑
   b) If no to (a), is this due to:-
       i) recent surgery?   ☑   ☐
      ii) trauma to limbs?   ☐   ☐
     iii) pain from wound?   ☐   ☐
      iv) a long term problem?   ☑   ☐
   c) Can it be improved to a limited extent?   ☑   ☐
   d) Drugs - is the patient taking i) steroids?   ☐   ☑
                                   ii) anti-inflammatory
                                       drugs?   ☐   ☑

7. **Sleep**

   a) Is the patient able to sleep for long periods at
      night time?   ☐   ☑
   b) If no to (a), is this due to pain?   ☑   ☐

8. **Underlying Disease**

   a) Is there underlying disease present?   ☑   ☐
   b) If yes to (a), please state. Gall bladder disease
   c) Is it in its terminal stages?   ☐   ☐

9. **Medical Intervention**

   a) Is patient taking cytotoxic drugs?   ☐   ☑
   b) Has patient recently undergone a course of
      radiotherapy?   ☐   ☑

CD/MH 17.12.87

SPECIFIC ASSESSMENT FOR A PATIENT WITH SUTURED INCISION/LACERATION

Name: Cynthia SMITH

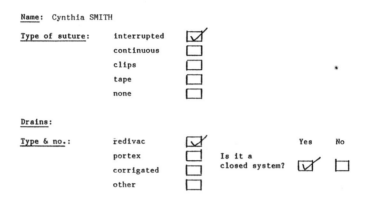

Type of suture: interrupted ☑
                 continuous   ☐
                 clips   ☐
                 tape   ☐
                 none   ☐

Drains:

Type & no.: redivac   ☑   Yes   No
             portex   ☐   Is it a
             corrigated ☐   closed system?   ☑   ☐
             other   ☐

Wound appearance - Location Midline abdominal incision

Date										
	Yes	No	Yes	No	Yes	No	Yes	No	Yes	No
Clean and dry		✓	✓		✓					
Localised tenderness		✓	✓		✓					
Swelling of incision line	✓		✓		✓					
Redness of incision line more than 1 cm		✓			✓	✓				
Localised heat		✓	✓		✓					
Purulent drainage		✓	✓		✓					
Approximation of skin edges	✓		✓		✓					
Serosanguinous drainage	✓		✓		✓					

Suggested Plan:

● *Nursing interventions* ●

Problem	Plan	Rationale
(1) Wound infection	(a) Remove 2–3 sutures over reddened area.	Allows free drainage of any pus.
Goal Resolve infection, promote healing.	(b) Insert sinus forceps into wound to expedite drainage.	
	(c) Take bacterial swab of fluid.	To identify infecting bacteria.
	(d) Irrigate opened area with warm sterile saline.	To assist drainage of pus.
	(e) Apply low-adherent dressing and absorbent pads, tape into position.	To protect wound and absorb drainage.
	(f) Change dressing daily or when strike through occurs.	Sodden dressings provide pathway for bacteria.
	(g) Monitor temperature 4 hrly.	Pyrexia indicates infection.
(2) Obesity	(a) 1000 kcal diet provided by dietitian.	To continue weight loss.
Goal Continue weight loss of 1 kg/week.	(b) Encourage Mrs Smith to persevere with diet.	Many dieters become despondent and/or bored.

● *Evaluation* ●

Problem	Evaluation
(1) Wound infection	A further 2 sutures were removed in order to allow complete drainage of infected material. The cavity was irrigated twice daily and a new dressing applied. By the eighth postoperative day, the drainage of pus was minimal and the cavity appeared clean. A Silastic foam stent ™ was inserted and Mrs Smith taught how to care for it herself. She was discharged home to care for the wound under the supervision of the community nurse.
(2) Obesity	In view of the excessive discharge from the wound, Mrs Smith's diet was changed to 1500 Kcal daily with a high protein content. She was to return to the previous dietary restrictions after discharge from hospital.

7.3 CARE OF A PATIENT WITH A PRESSURE SORE

7.3.1 Background information

Mr Samuel Jones is 66 years old. He fell over whilst gardening and sustained a fractured neck of femur. He lay injured for three hours after his fall as his wife was out. He suffers from rheumatoid arthritis and takes Ibuprofen as medication.

● *Patient assessment* ●

ASSESSMENT FORM FOR PATIENTS WITH OPEN WOUNDS/MAJOR SURGERY

Name: Samuel JONES   **Hospital No.:** 23456
Ward: 3   **Consultant:** Mr Benn
Age: 66 yrs   **Sex:** M   **Waterlow Score:** 20
Date of Assessment: 17 April

15 April: Pin-and-Plate operation for fracture neck of femur.

		Yes	No
1.	Maintaining a Safe Environment		
	Infection		
	a) Is infection present elsewhere (ie not the wound)?	☐	☑
	b) If yes to (a), is this being treated?	☐	☐
2.	Communicating		
	a) Are there any communication problems?	☐	☑
	b) If yes to (a), please specify.		
	c) Does patient appear anxious?	☐	☑
	d) HAD score =		
3.	Breathing		
	a) Has the patient known cardiovascular disease?	☐	☑
	b) Is peripheral vascular disease present?	☐	☑
	c) Is oedema present?	☐	☑
	d) Is there discoloration of the legs?	☐	☑
	e) Is the patient anaemic? Don't know ☐	☐	☑
	f) If yes to (e), is this being treated?	☐	☐
4.	Eating and Drinking		
	Nutritional Status		
	a) Is the patient eating a well balanced diet?	☑	☐
	Comments:		
	b) Are there signs of i) obesity?	☐	☑
	ii) emaciation?	☐	☑
	iii) muscle wasting?	☐	☐
	c) Is weight within 'normal' limits?	☑	☐
	d) Has patient lost weight recently?	☐	☑
	Comments:		
	e) Are plasma proteins low? Don't know ☐	☐	☐
	Other comments: NOTE - Check weight on 20 April		
	Underlying Disease		
	a) Is the patient a diabetic?	☐	☑
	b) If yes to (a), is it stable at present?	☐	☐
	Smoking		
	a) Does the patient smoke?	☑	☐
	b) If yes to (a), is it - 0 - 20/day	☐	
	20 - 40/day	☐	
	40 - 60/day	☐	
	60 + /day	☐	
	SMokes 1 pipe/day		

- 2 -

	Yes	No

5. Eliminating

a) Is the patient incontinent of i) urine? — No ✓
   ii) faeces? — No ✓
b) If yes to (a), can the problem be improved?
   Comments:
c) Has the patient uraemia?
d) Is the blood urea above 7mmol/l?
   Don't know ☐

6. Mobilising

a) Is the patient fully mobile? — No ✓
b) If no to (a), is this due to:-
   i) recent surgery? — Yes ✓
   ii) trauma to limbs? — Yes ✓
   iii) pain from wound?
   iv) a long term problem?
c) Can it be improved to a limited extent? — Yes ✓
d) Drugs - is the patient taking i) steroids?
   ii) anti-inflammatory drugs? — Yes ✓

7. Sleep

a) Is the patient able to sleep for long periods at
   night time? 2 hrly turning disturbs him - now reduced — No ✓
b) If no to (a), is this due to pain? — No ✓

8. Underlying Disease

a) Is there underlying disease present? — Yes ✓
b) If yes to (a), please state. rheumatoid arthritis
c) Is it in its terminal stages? — No ✓

9. Medical Intervention

a) Is patient taking cytotoxic drugs? — No ✓
b) Has patient recently undergone a course of
   radiotherapy? — No ✓

CD/HH 17.12.87

SPECIFIC ASSESSMENT FOR A PATIENT WITH PRESSURE SORES

Name: Samuel JONES   Waterlow Score: 20

                                       Date: 17 April

Position of Sore:

(sacrum)   R   L   R   L   R   L   Other
             Buttocks   Trochanter   Heels

Grade: 3

Support System: Nimbus

Lifting/Turning Regime: 3-4 hrly

Description of Sore(s): (if more than one sore add further boxes and
                          label according to position)

Deep   ☑

Shallow   ☐

Necrotic   ☑ Patchy

Clinically infected ☐

Sloughy   ☐

Granulating   ☐

Epithelialising   ☐

Offensive smell   ☐

Heavy exudate   ☑

Size in cm 3 x 2 cm
            2.6 cm deep

Suggested Plan:

Comments

Sam lay for approximately 3 hrs after his fall.

Operating time 1½ hrs.

● *Nursing interventions* ●

Problem	Plan	Rationale
(1) Potential problem: wound infection. *Goal* Early detection of infection.	(a) Observe wound daily for evidence of infection or haematoma. Report any redness, swelling or undue pain to the nurse in charge. (b) Record temperature 4 hrly.	This will ensure early detection of any infection. Infection may cause pyrexia.
(2) Pressure sore on sacrum *Goal* Promote rapid healing by second intention.	(a) Clean sore by irrigation using warm saline. (b) Apply Intrasite Gel ™ by squeezing a layer 1 cm thick onto a Melolin ™ pad. Apply to wound and cover with absorbent pad, tape in position. (c) Change dressing daily until all necrotic tissue is removed, then every three days. (d) Measure diameter and depth of sore 2 × weekly. (e) Place patient on a Nimbus ™ mattress. (f) Turn patient 4–6 hrly when in bed. (g) Use a suitable height chair with a 3″ foam cushion. Encourage Mr Jones to stand for 1 minute every hour.	Reduces trauma to wound. Maintains moist environment. Encourages autolysis of necrotic tissue. Provides objective record. Provides pressure relief. Less disturbance of sleep at night. Provides pressure relief. Allows blood to flow into tissues compressed by sitting.

● *Evaluation* ●

Problem	Evaluation
(1) Potential problem: wound infection	No evidence of infection.
(2) Pressure sore on sacrum	Once the necrotic tissue was removed, the sore was found to be larger than the initial assessment suggested. It healed slowly and delayed Mr Jones' expected discharge date by a week.

7.4 CARE OF A PATIENT WITH LEG ULCERS

7.4.1 Background information

Miss Alice Black is 77 years old. She lives alone except for her cat. She has had a leg ulcer for 10 months and has difficulty doing her shopping. As a result, her nutritional status is poor. She had in any case lost interest in food since the death of her sister 3 years ago. She has no other near relatives. Miss Black has been admitted to hospital because her ulcer has become acutely infected, with cellulitis in the tissues around it. She was reluctant to come into hospital and very anxious about her cat which she has never left before. The district nurse persuaded her it was necessary to be admitted and arranged for a neighbour to care for the cat.

● *Patient assessment* ●

ASSESSMENT FORM FOR PATIENTS WITH OPEN WOUNDS/MAJOR SURGERY

Name: Miss Alice BLACK   **Hospital No.:** 12345

Ward: 6   **Consultant:** Dr Brown

Age: 77 yrs   **Sex:** F   **Waterlow Score:** 12

Date of Assessment: 2 September

Admitted with cellulitis around venous ulcer L leg

1. <u>Maintaining a Safe Environment</u>   Yes   No

    <u>Infection</u>

    a) Is infection present elsewhere (ie not the wound)?   ☐   ☑
    b) If yes to (a), is this being treated?   ☐   ☐

2. <u>Communicating</u>

    a) Are there any communication problems?   ☐   ☑
    b) If yes to (a), please specify.
    c) Does patient appear anxious?   ☑   ☐
    d) HAD score = very worried about leaving cat

3. <u>Breathing</u>

    a) Has the patient known cardiovascular disease?   ☐   ☑
    b) Is peripheral vascular disease present?   ☐   ☑
    c) Is oedema present?   ☑   ☐
    d) Is there discoloration of the legs?   ☑   ☐
    e) Is the patient anaemic?   Don't know   ☐   ☐   ☑
    f) If yes to (e), is this being treated?

4. <u>Eating and Drinking</u>

    <u>Nutritional Status</u>

    a) Is the patient eating a well balanced diet?   ☐   ☑
       Comments:
    b) Are there signs of i) obesity?   ☐   ☑
                         ii) emaciation?   ☐   ☑
                        iii) muscle wasting?   ☐   ☑
    c) Is weight within 'normal' limits?   ☐   ☑
    d) Has patient lost weight recently? Wt: 49 kg   ☑   ☐
       Comments:
    e) Are plasma proteins low?   Don't know   ☑   ☐   ☐
       Other comments: Difficulty in getting to shops, seems
       to eat little protein or fresh fruit or vegetables.
    <u>Underlying Disease</u>

    a) Is the patient a diabetic?   ☐   ☑
    b) If yes to (a), is it stable at present?   ☐   ☐

    <u>Smoking</u>

    a) Does the patient smoke?   ☐   ☑
    b) If yes to (a), is it - 0 - 20/day
                          20 - 40/day
                          40 - 60/day
                          60 +   /day

- 2 -

	Yes	No

5. Eliminating

a) Is the patient incontinent of i) urine? ☐ ☑

                ii) faeces? ☐ ☑

b) If yes to (a), can the problem be improved? ☐ ☐

   Comments:

c) Has the patient uraemia? ☐ ☐

d) Is the blood urea above 7mmol/l? ☐ ☐

               Don't know ☐ ☐ ☐

6. Mobilising

a) Is the patient fully mobile? ☐ ☑

b) If no to (a), is this due to:-

   i) recent surgery? ☐ ☐

   ii) trauma to limbs? ☐ ☐

   iii) pain from wound? ☑ ☐

   iv) a long term problem? ☐ ☐

c) Can it be improved to a limited extent? ☑ ☐

d) Drugs - is the patient taking i) steroids? ☐ ☐

                ii) anti-inflammatory
                   drugs? ☐ ☐

7. Sleep

a) Is the patient able to sleep for long periods at
   night time? ☐ ☑

b) If no to (a), is this due to pain? ☑ ☐

   Recent sensation of throbbing in L leg.

8. Underlying Disease

a) Is there underlying disease present? ☑ ☐

b) If yes to (a), please state. Venous ulcer L leg

c) Is it in its terminal stages? (history of DVT) ☐ ☑

9. Medical Intervention

a) Is patient taking cytotoxic drugs? ☐ ☑

b) Has patient recently undergone a course of
   radiotherapy? ☐ ☑

CD/MH 17.12.87

SPECIFIC ASSESSMENT FOR PATIENT WITH LEG ULCER OR FOOT ULCER

Name: Alice BLACK   **Date:** 2 September   **Ward:**

Type of Ulcer:		Appearance of leg:			Associated Problems
Venous	☑	oedema	☑	warm/~~cold~~	
Arterial	☐	discoloured	☑	pedal pulses	
Mix ed	☐	white & shiny	☐	R✓ L✓	
Neuropathic	☐				

Description of Ulcer(s):

necrotic	☐	epithelialising	☐
clinically infected	☑	heavy exudate	☑
sloughy	☐	offensive smell	☑
granulating	☐	Size in cm	.....

Indicate position on diagram below:

R   L

LAT   MED   MED   LAT

R   L   L   R

Area of cellulit-is

Suggested Plan

Leg measurements

R	calf	26 cm
	ankle	14 cm
L	calf	30 cm
	ankle	20 cm

• *Nursing interventions* •

Problem	Plan	Rationale
(1) Infected leg ulcer	(a) Wound swab to be taken.	To identify infecting bacteria and suitable antibiotics.
Goal To reduce infection so Miss Black can return home.	(b) Bathe leg daily in foot bath using warm water.	Helps to remove skin scales. Improves morale as patient feels clean.
	(c) Apply Iodosorb™ ointment to a depth of 5 mm over ulcer. Cover with non-adherent dressing and absorbent pads. Change daily. Change outer pads more frequently if strikethrough occurs.	Iodine is a broad-spectrum antiseptic. Patient has no known allergy to iodine. Sodden dressings provide a pathway for bacteria.
	(d) Make a tracing of ulcer and repeat weekly.	To provide objective measurement.
	(e) Bed rest except for toilet and dressing change.	Rest promotes tissue regeneration.
(2) Oedema left leg *Goal* To reduce oedema so that left leg measures the same as right leg.	(a) Position patient so that feet are higher than heart for periods of 1–2 hrs 3 × daily.	It is unrealistic to expect anyone to stay in this position constantly. It is better to set realistic targets.
	(b) Provide a chart for patient to keep her own record (see Fig. 5.11).	This will help to involve Miss Black in her own care and set a precedent for when she returns home.
(3) Venous insufficiency *Goal* To maximize venous return.	(a) Apply Tensopress™ bandage as a support bandage from toe to knee. Reapply daily, using new bandages as necessary.	Graduated compression improves venous return. Bandages eventually lose their elasticity.
	(b) Order a below knee Class II support stocking.	Stockings provide more effective graduated compression.
	(c) Teach Miss Black leg and feet exercises and supervise 2 × daily.	Stimulates drainage of calf muscle pump.
(4) Poor diet *Goal* Miss Black will take at least 1500 kcal daily including protein and fresh fruit	(a) Arrange for dietitian to talk to Miss Black about her dietary needs.	Miss Black needs education as to her dietary requirements.
	(b) Assist in selecting suitable menus.	
	(c) A small glass of sherry to be given each day before lunch.	Stimulates appetite.
(5) Anxiety about cat *Goal* To alleviate anxiety concerning cat.	(a) Allow Miss Black to talk about her cat and to express her anxieties.	Expression of feelings and anxieties alleviates stress.
	(b) Find out 'phone number of neighbour and arrange for Miss Black to ring regularly.	Regular reassurance about her cat's condition.
(6) Pain from infected ulcer *Goal* The patient will say she is pain-free.	(a) Give prescribed analgesia as required and monitor effectiveness. Ensure adequate analgesia is given at night-time.	Pain disturbs rest and reduces feelings of well being.

• *Evaluation* •

Problem	Evaluation
(1) Leg ulcer	The cellulitis subsided after a course of antibiotics and the use of Iodosorb ™. By 10 days there was evidence of granulation and a considerable reduction in exudate. The dressing was changed to Granuflex ™. On discharge home, the patient will attend clinic weekly and the district nurse will be asked to assess for further visits.
(2) Oedema left leg	The oedema had considerably reduced, but left leg remained slightly larger than the right. Miss Black to continue to elevate her legs at home, using the chart.
(3) Venous insufficiency	Miss Black was able to wear her compression stocking. The nurses showed her the easiest way to put it on. She has become confident doing the leg and foot exercises and her mobility is slightly improved.
(4) Poor diet	Appetite now much improved. Miss Black has become aware of the need for a varied diet. Help arranged with shopping.
(5) Anxiety about cat	Miss Black has been reassured by reports about her cat. She is looking forward to returning home.
(6) Pain from infected ulcer	As the infection subsided, so did the pain. Miss Black now says she has no pain and is sleeping better.

Chapter 8
Conclusions

8.1 INTRODUCTION

This chapter seeks to address several issues related to wound care. Some of them do not fall readily into the other chapters, others consider the future rather than the present. Some of the issues, may be described as contentious, and although it is intended to provide a rounded view of the specific issue, the conclusions are those of the author.

8.2 THE COST OF HEALING

The emphasis so far in this book has been to consider wound care without reference to the cost involved. Much attention has been given to the modern products and the research supporting their use. Although there is little doubt as to the efficacy of these dressings, their use is by no means universal. One of the reasons may be cost.

Generally, when a product is chosen to dress a wound, little attention is paid to the cost of the materials being used. However, it has to be pointed out that the *choice* of dressings is often limited because of cost. The decision regarding the particular products to be made available may be made by non-clinicians without reference to the user. There is an increasing interest in cost-effective care and the use of audit. Nurses need to become aware of the cost of the care they give so that they can argue their case effectively for quality of care. This should not just be limited to the basic cost of dressings – although it does have a part to play – but should also look at the wider issues.

8.2.1 The cost of materials

Many of the second generation dressings are considerably more expensive than the traditional dressings that they have replaced. A piece of gauze costs a few pence, whereas the new dressings can cost in the region of £1–£2 for a 10 × 10 cm size. Inevitably, there has been resistance to their introduction on grounds of cost. But the major advantage of these dressings is that they do not require daily changing and they may well speed up the healing process – and, overall, cost less in terms of nursing time.

A study by Davis (1988) found the cost of five month's traditional treatment for one patient with a leg ulcer to be £868.47. During the following five months a hydrocolloid was used at the cost of £369.18. Not only did this represent a considerable saving, but the ulcer was healed as well! In another study, Johnson (1985) cites the case of a patient with a leg ulcer which had been dressed daily for seven years at a cost of about £6000. It was healed in under seven months at a cost of £430 using a modern dressing.

It is relatively easy to calculate the cost of materials required to treat a wound for a week. The following equation can be used:

$$\text{Cost of materials} \times \text{Number of dressing changes per week}$$

Table 8.1 demonstrates the costings for a number of dressings. It clearly shows that the use of modern products is cost effective. Anyone can undertake a similar exercise to cost the dressings being used in their area. The costings should include all materials required at each dressing change. This might be dressing packs, lotions, gloves, the actual dressing and anything else that is needed.

8.2.2 A wound management policy

There is a huge range of dressings available today. It is, therefore, irresponsible to argue for a total freedom of choice in all areas. It makes sense for hospitals and health authorities to have a policy in regard to the range of dressings available. The selection of dressings should include an example from each of the following:

- Alginate dressing
- Bead dressing
- Charcoal dressing
- Foam dressing
- Hydrocolloid
- Hydrogel

Table 8.1 Cost comparisons of several dressings.

Dressing type	Dressing change	Weekly cost
Gauze + Pad	Daily	£6.16
Jelonet™ 10 × 10 cm	Daily	£6.72
Granuflex™ 10 × 10 cm	2 × weekly	£5.92
Inadine™ 9.5 × 9.5 cm	4 × weekly	£4.12
Lyofoam™ 10 × 10 cm	3 × weekly	£4.59
Opsite Flexigrid™ 10 × 12 cm	2 × weekly	£3.26
Intrasite Gel™ 25 g sachet	3 × weekly	£7.38
Sorbsan™ 10 × 10 cm	2 × weekly	£3.98
Gauze Packing	Daily	£12.39
Gauze Packing	8 hourly	£37.17
Silastic™ Foam	New stent weekly	£9.75
Sorbsan Packing™	3 × weekly	£15.03

NB The dressings used are only examples of modern products and do not imply that any others are not also cost effective.

- Paste bandage
- Vapour permeable film

A very important aspect is to have a good range of sizes: a dressing may be ineffective because the wrong size has been used.

Any policy needs to be reviewed regularly. There are new dressings being launched all the time. Each one should be adequately evaluated in the clinical area. If there is a clinical nurse specialist in post, she/he is the ideal person to coordinate such work. Many policies are prepared in the form of a small booklet for distribution to the clinical areas, possibly with supporting wall posters.

In the community the Drug Tariff restricts the selection of dressings. As yet there is not a full range of products available for the community nurse. Another problem is the limited range of sizes available; most of them are small sizes. This may be a false economy as several dressings may be required to cover a wound, costing more than a larger size dressing.

8.2.3 Nursing time

There is not a great deal published in relation to the cost of nursing time. What little there is concentrates on community costs, where the cost of each visit has been calculated. The costs vary considerably from £8 to £25 depending on the area. Unpublished data (Milward, 1988) showed that improved wound management reduced visits to patients for the purpose of dressing changes. A study of 26 patients over a period of three months found that the number of visits was reduced by 990, at a saving of around £14 500 for both visits and materials.

It is extremely difficult to consider the time saving benefits in the hospital setting. It is easy to brush this aside with comments such as 'the nurses have to be there anyway'. Many complicated dressings can take up to an hour to perform. If this can be reduced by changing the dressing on alternate days, a saving of three or four hours per week could be made. Less frequent dressing changes would lead to even greater savings, thus leaving the nurse more time to talk to the patients or to encourage a better fluid or dietary intake – care which otherwise may be neglected due to lack of time.

8.2.4 Cost to the hospital

The cost to the hospital has to be considered in terms of delayed healing or complications delaying recovery. Two areas which can be considered are pressure sores and surgical wound infection. Much work has been undertaken looking at the prevention and management of pressure sores. One classic study by Hibbs (1988) calculated the cost of treating a patient with a grade 4 pressure sore which developed as a complication of hip surgery. Every cost was included, such as nursing time, catering costs, domestic services, x-rays and so on. The patient was in hospital for 180 days at a total cost of £25 905.58. Further calculations showed that the money spent treating this patient would have paid for 20 standard cases. In the time that the bed was 'blocked' a further 16 hip or knee replacements could have been undertaken. A very good argument for prevention rather than cure.

With the increase in litigation, some patients have taken action against a health authority for the development of a pressure sore. The first litigant was awarded £98 000 damages (Robertson, 1984). Others have followed. Health authorities are gradually coming to terms with the fact that inadequate mattresses whose foam has collapsed and insufficient pressure relieving equipment is negligence in the eyes of the law (Livesley & Simpson, 1989).

Surgical audit is a useful way of counting the cost of wound infection post-operatively. Cruse & Foord (1980) found that postoperative wound infection increased patient hospitalization by an average of 10.1 days. This was costed at more than $2000 for the hospital bed alone. Green and Wenzel (1977) undertook a controlled study comparing length of stay and costs between surgical patients who developed infection and those who did not. They found a considerable increase in length of stay and cost in those patients with infection. Extended stay inevitably results in cancelled admissions and increased waiting lists. This may result in loss of regional funding or loss of business.

8.2.5 Cost to the patient

For the many people suffering from chronic wounds there is no way their pain and suffering can be quantified, or the effect it has on their quality of life. Leg ulcers are classic examples. The patient may have restricted mobility as a result of the ulcers. If he or she lives alone, it may mean it is difficult to get to the shops. This may lead to a poor diet which will affect the ability to heal the ulcer. Another problem may be pain at night which encourages the patient to sleep in an armchair with the legs hanging down. As a result stasis oedema may develop with the risk of thrombosis or heart failure.

Social isolation is another aspect of unrecognized cost to many people. Many patients are very conscious of the odour from their wounds and so refuse to go out. For others, sadly, the nurse dressing their ulcer may be the only real contact with the outside world. One small study found that those patients with the lowest number of social contacts were those whose ulcers recurred within a six month period (Wise, 1986). So, for those people, the cost of healing was actually social isolation.

The cost to a younger person is not only in pain, but also in loss of earnings which may cause considerable hardship. It may also affect future employment. There is disruption of family life; even visiting hospital may be difficult for the partner if there are young children in the family. It should also be remembered that there is still a mortality risk from postoperative complications following any surgery.

8.2.6 Cost to the community

The idea that poorly healing wounds have a cost to the community is one that has not really been explored. An infected wound not only causes unnecessary pain and suffering to the patient and delays discharge from hospital – it also means a loss of productive work. A person's labour not only earns money for the labourer, but is also a benefit to the community in terms of goods produced or services rendered. If this is lost through incapacity, then the cost is not only that of the loss but also of the cost of sickness benefit. This is not to say that such rights should not be available, indeed they should, but their cost should be recognized.

8.2.7 Conclusion

So what is the true cost of healing? It is obvious that there is no easy answer. It is most certainly more than comparing the cost of a piece of gauze with a film dressing. The *Code of Conduct* exhorts nurses always to act so as to 'serve the interests of society, and above all to safeguard the interests of individual patients and clients' (UKCC, 1992). Among other things surely that means that quality of care is paramount.

As the use of various types of audit becomes a more frequent part of hospital life, an opportunity is provided to demonstrate that *quality of care can be cost effective*. There *is* a case for adequate prevention of both pressure sores and post-operative wound infection as well as appropriate wound management. Nurses should be there to see that the hospital does the patient no harm.

This following section is based on an article which appeared in *Nursing* (Dealey, C. (1990) *Nursing* **4**: 15, 14–16) and is reproduced by kind permission of the publishers.

8.3 NURSES AND THEIR ROLE IN WOUND CARE

Nurses have an important role to play in wound management and need to be aware of their responsibilities. Obviously this role must be seen in the context of the multidisciplinary team, as the wounds cannot be seen in isolation from the rest of the body. However, many different medical specialities are also involved in wound care, so the constituent members may vary according to the needs of the patient. In many areas, multidisciplinary teams are preparing policies in relation to wound management and pressure sore prevention. Such efforts are to be applauded as they can make major improvements to the standards of patient care.

8.3.1 Accountability

The UKCC Code of Professional Conduct (UKCC, 1992a) states that nurses are accountable for their actions. Ralph (1989) suggested that professional accountability is an obligation on the practitioner that binds her/him to a code of conduct which is based on the expectations of society that each nurse will use her/his discretion and skill to safeguard her/his patients and act in every way to uphold professional standards. It must also be emphasized that the prescriptive authority that doctors have over nurses does not absolve nurses from the consequences of their actions. If a doctor prescribes an inappropriate dosage of a drug which is then administered by a nurse, the nurse also has to accept responsibility and be accountable for her/his actions.

The document *Exercising Accountability*, (UKCC, 1989) defines the responsibilities of the accountable nurse. Most of these can be related to the nurse caring for a patient with a wound. They can be summarised as to:

- Promote and safeguard the interests of the patient.
- Have concern for the environment of care.
- Have concern that the patient is enabled to give informed consent.
- Be an advocate for the patient.
- Work in collaboration and co-operation within the health care team.
- Make known any objection to participation in care.

The foremost responsibility for the nurse is always to promote and safeguard the interests of the patient.

One aspect of that is that the practitioner should seek to achieve high standards of care. The *Strategy for Nursing*, (DOH, 1990) clearly states that such care should be firmly based on research. When this principle is applied to wound care, it means that the nurse caring for a patient with a wound has the responsibility to be knowledgeable about current research and its implications for practice as well as how to actually apply the dressing. There should be a rationale for the dressing selection. Dressings should not be chosen for reasons such as 'We always do it this way here', or 'I have used this dressing for the last 30 years, why should I change?'. Decisions should be based on a proper assessment of the wound.

A further responsibility for the nurse is that of highlighting inadequate provision of care. Inadequate provision of care is seen as negligence in law (Livesley & Simpson, 1989). This can be related to matters such as an insufficient supply of pressure-relieving equipment. The nurse should be prepared to make representation to a higher authority and, most importantly, make accurate records of what the consequences might be for the patient without the equipment.

The Patient's Charter (Deptartment of Health, 1991), states that all patients have the right to a clear explanation of any proposed treatment. All aspects of wound management should be explained to the patient. For example, several of the interactive dressings change their appearance or produce a distinctive odour on removal. This may cause anxiety to the patient unless a full explanation has been given.

Advocacy on behalf of a patient has many aspects. It should not be seen as confrontational, but as a constructive activity. This involves working in co-operation and collaboration with other healthcare professionals and may also involve entering into informed debate on the value or otherwise of specific forms of treatment. This also relates to objection to participation in care and treatment. Most frequently, the issue being debated seems to be the use of antiseptic solutions. Many nurses object to their use because of the research demonstrating their harmful properties. The doctor concerned may see this as an attempt to usurp his/her power. Walsh & Ford (1989) have discussed some of these aspects of the nurse/doctor relationship. Certainly, decision making in wound care seems to be an area of dispute.

8.3.2 Decision-making in wound care

Any discussion of the role of the nurse in wound care has to consider the relationship between medicine and nursing. There is considerable overlap between the knowledge base of the two professions. Nurses and doctors can be described as key players in the field of treatment and care of patients (RCN, 1990). There is no clear-cut division of responsibility between the two. Instead there is a need to work together in harmony.

An essential aspect of wound management is assessment of the wound and planning appropriate treatment. There has been much discussion as to who should make these decisions – the nurse or the doctor. Sutton & Wallace (1990) interviewed 66 doctors who were either senior registrars or consultants from both the departments of surgery and the care of the elderly in one health authority. Although 85% considered that pressure sores required a team approach, 82% relied on nurses to choose the topical agent to be applied to a sore.

A very small study was carried out by Chandler (1990) who interviewed both nurses and doctors on two surgical wards. She found that the nurses had a far greater awareness of current research and modern products than the doctors. However, despite this, they still relied on the doctors to determine the dressing to be used. The doctor's choice was mostly based on preference or habit.

Gwyther (1988) questioned 85 student and qualified nurses regarding wound care practices. One question addressed the issue of decision-making. Some 83.5% felt it was a sister or staff nurse who chose the dressing to be used whereas 45.9% suggested that the decision was made by a doctor. No specific type of wound was indicated in the question. It should also be noted that 92.9% of the respondents said that they had been taught about wound assessment.

Flanagan (1992) interviewed 24 qualified nurses about their views on wound care. They were all aware of the the clinical factors which influence dressing selection. However, they tended to be more interested in discussing the influence of the medical staff on dressing choice. Many expressed anxiety about the differences of opinion which arose between the two disciplines. They also described the types of manipulative behaviour that could be displayed by both nurses and doctors. There seemed to be some inconsistency between specialist areas. Nurses in medical areas, intensive care units and accident and emergency departments were more likely to be able to select treatments than those working in surgical wards.

These studies highlight several issues:

(1) Nurses seem to make most of the decisions in relation to pressure sore management - possibly because pressure sores have traditionally been seen as a nursing problem.

(2) Surgeons inevitably seem to have a greater interest in choosing dressings, seeing the surgical wound as their responsibility.

(3) Although research into wound management has had a high profile in nursing journals, this has not been so in medical journals.

(4) The fact that nurses actually carry out the dressing change means that they have more confidence in their use and mode of action than their medical

colleagues. This is particularly of relevance when using interactive wound management products.

(5) There are many anecdotal reports of conflict between nurses and doctors over what constitutes an appropriate dressing. It should also be noted that often nurses will carry out medical prescription even if they do not believe it is appropriate. Gilchrist (1989) argues that the UKCC have not provided clear guidelines in this respect. Whilst stating that the nurse should question the use of substances that may be harmful, it does not say clearly whether the nurse should still carry out the treatment, once she has raised her objections, if the substance has been charted on the prescription sheet.

Many nurses believe that they should automatically have the right to choose a suitable dressing for the patient, and in practice many actually make that decision. In short, having the right to select a dressing can be seen as one aspect of autonomy, or freedom to act. Vaughan (1989) suggests that autonomy is not complete freedom, but 'freedom to act within the bounds of competence, which are in turn confined by the boundaries of knowledge'. No nurse should be seeking such autonomy unless she/he has sufficient knowledge and competence for the task in hand. The discussions related to the right of the community nurse to prescribe a limited range of products has heightened awareness of the importance of education and training. Autonomy and accountability carry responsibilities. The document *The Scope of Professional Practice* (UKCC, 1992b) states the principles that must be maintained within nursing practice. They include honestly acknowledging the limits of personal skills and knowledge as well as ensuring that any extension of professional practice always conforms to the *Code of Practice*.

It must always be remembered that the wound cannot be treated in isolation; it is, after all, attached to a patient. Medical intervention may well be needed for effective treatment. For example, vascular surgery may be necessary for ischaemic ulcers to heal. There are many examples where nursing and medicine complement each other and it is important for each discipline to have respect for the other.

8.3.3 The nursing process

Assessment and planning

Assessment of the patient and the wound should be carried out and recorded in a methodical manner. In 1993, the UKCC produced the document *Standards for Records and Record Keeping*. Records are perceived to be an integral and essential part of care allowing good communication between professionals. Assessment may reveal the need to involve other members of the multidisciplinary team in the care of the patient. In the case of patients at risk of developing pressure sores or those already suffering from them, specialist equipment may be required. The nurse has a major role in planning these aspects of care and in co-ordinating the input from other members of the team. Thus, a coherent strategy can be established which maximises wound healing.

Implementation

Although there may be dispute over who assesses a wound and plans the care, there is none over implementation of the plan. The vast majority of wounds are dressed by nurses. Applying a dressing which is both comfortable and remains in place requires a degree of manual dexterity. Experience is also of considerable importance. An understanding of the action of the interactive wound management products is also necessary when removing the old dressing.

Evaluation

At each dressing change the nurse should monitor the progress of the wound and the effectiveness of the dressing. Evaluation is an ongoing process. Part of evaluation must also be documentation and communication with others. Effective documentation will record the size and appearance of the wound. Any changes need to be communicated to others as part of the exchange of information about patient progress.

8.3.4 Education

Another aspect of the role of the nurse in wound care is providing education to others. Patient education is important to enhance compliance and an understanding of different aspects of care. Nurses may also require information about any aspect of wound management. There is also a need to provide education for medical students and junior doctors. A survey by Bennet (1992) of medical undergraduate teaching on chronic wound care found that tuition ranged from 0 to 35.5 hours. It is already recognized that nurses teach junior doctors a great deal when they are first qualified; wound management is yet another topic which requires consideration.

8.3.5 Nurse specialist in wound care

A new nursing speciality developed in the late 1980s – that of the specialist in wound care. There are now between 50 and 100 nurse specialists in the UK. The precise number is difficult to determine as there is no formal register and the precise title may vary. The most frequently used are 'clincal nurse specialist in tissue viability' and 'wound care specialist'. As yet there is no formal qualification specific to wound care which would provide credence for the role, such as there are for infection control nurses or stoma nurses.

A major aspect of the role of the specialist is in providing expert advice on the management and prevention of wounds of all types. As well as having a good understanding of the range of wound management products, many of these specialist nurses are able to provide guidance on the selection of pressue-relieving mattresses and beds. The specialist may be called upon to negotiate with others in relation to the care that is needed for particular patients. Much of the clinical care that is given provides ideal teaching opportunities on a one-to-one basis. A number of nurse specialists are involved in wider teaching at study days and conferences.

Many hospitals and units are developing policies, such as standards with respect to wound management, formularies of wound management products, and strategies for pressure sore prevention. The wound care specialist can play an integral role in the development and implementation of such policies. Guidelines on pressure sore development which will shortly be published by the Department of Health recommend that each NHS Trust or other provider units should have access to a clinical nurse specialist in pressure sores.

Finally, many nurse specialists are involved in research in a whole range of aspects of wound healing. The include pressure sore prevalence and incidence monitoring, surveys of equipment, surveys of nursing practice, evaluations of products and equipment as well as aspects of cell biology.

8.3.6 Conclusions

Nurses have an important role to play in wound care as summarized in Fig. 8.1. However, they do not work in isolation and optimal care can only be provided in the context of the multidisciplinary team. Ultimately, nurses are accountable to their patients. In order to provide the highest standards of care, the nurse should ensure that she/he is aware of recent developments in the field and their implications for practice.

8.4 FUTURE TRENDS IN WOUND CARE

The changes and developments in the understanding of wound healing and the management of wounds have been immense in the last twenty years. It is interesting to postulate how dressings will develop in the future. Passive dressings were followed by interactive dressings. It has been suggested that interactive dressings would be followed by intelligent dressings. This name has been given to the concept of dressings that will respond to the amount of exudate produced by a wound by

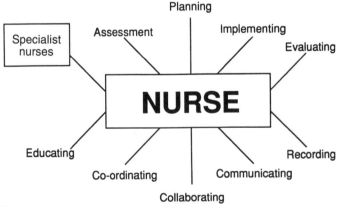

Fig. 8.1   The role of the nurse in wound care.

becoming more or less moisture vapour permeable. However, the area that has been arousing the greatest interest is that of growth factors.

Developments in molecular biology have made it possible to identify a range of biological mediators which have a highly complex role in tissue repair. Sporn & Roberts (1988) suggest that it would be better to refer to them as multifunctional peptides rather than growth factors. But whatever name is gven to them, their precise mode of action is still imperfectly understood.

Around 30 growth factors have been identified. Turner (1992) suggested that there are six principal growth factors. They are: platelet-derived growth factor (PDGF), epidermal growth factor (EGF), transforming growth factors alpha and beta (TGF-α and TGF-β), interleukin-1 (IL-1), fibroblast growth factor (FGF), and tumour necrosis factor alpha (TNF-α). Table 8.2 lists their actions.

The relevance of growth factors to tissue repair is two-fold. First, they obviously play an important role in normal wound healing; second, they have the potential to be used as a topical treatment to a wound in order to promote healing. A number of animal studies have demonstrated the effectiveness of growth factors used either in isolation or in combination (Greenhalgh *et al*, 1990; Lawrence *et al.*, 1986). There has been more difficulty in carrying out clinical trials. Falanga (1992) suggests that there are several reasons for this: more rigorous regulations have to be observed for use on humans; the cost of research is very expensive; it has been difficult to find a reliable agent to deliver the growth factors to the wound surface; initial results have not been as good as expected.

Some studies have shown promise, but have not provided hard evidence of the effectiveness of growth factors. Brown *et al.* (1991) used EGF on nine patients with chronic wounds in an uncontrolled trial and found some encouraging results. Robson *et al.* (1992) carried out a randomized double-blind placebo controlled trial

Table 8.2 Growth factors and their action in wound healing.

PDGF	Released from platelets during clotting. A vasoconstrictor, chemotactic for fibroblasts, monocytes (macrophages) and neutrophils. Plays role in development of granulation tissue.
EGF	Present in most body fluids. Increases proliferation of keratinocytes, endothelial cells, fibroblasts and others.
TGF-α	Stimulates mitogenesis of epithelial cells, keratinocyte migration and angiogenesis.
TGF-β	An immunosuppressive agent, stimulates fibroblasts and, possibly PDGF.
IL-1	Early host defence factor, released after injury; also stimulates proliferation of keratinocytes, endothelial cells and vascular smooth muscle cells. Chemotactic to monocytes, lymphocytes, neutrophils and keratinocytes.
FGF	Encourages cartilage repair, controls the differing proportions of collagen being produced.
TNF-α	Cytotoxic to tumour cells, activates neutrophils, macrophages and lymphocytes, mediator for resorption of cartilage and bone.

using PDGF on patients with pressure sores. Some 20 patients were entered into the trial and allocated to one of four groups using different doses of PDGF or the placebo. Those having the highest dose had a better healing response than the placebo group. However, the numbers of subjects in each group were too small for this to carry real weight.

There are still questions to be answered in relation to the use of growth factors. Their precise action needs to be understood. To use them effectively as a treatment the dosage of each factor, the appropriate combination and the method of delivery needs to be resolved. Eventually, their use may revolutionize wound healing, particularly in chronic wounds.

REFERENCES

Bennet, G. (1992) Medical undergraduate teaching in chronic wound care (a survey). *Journal of Tissue Viability* **2**: 2, 50–51.

Brown, G.L., Curtsinger, L., Jurkiewicz, M.J., Nahai, F. & Schultz, G. (1991) Stimulation of healing of chronic wounds by epidermal growth factor. *Plastic Reconstructive Surgery* **88**, 189–94.

Chandler, S. (1990) Wound management in surgical wards. *Nursing Times* **86**: 27, 54.

Cruse, P. & Foord, R. (1980) The epidemiology of wound infection: a ten-year prospective study of 62,939 wounds. *Surgical Clinics of North America* **60**: 1, 27–39.

Davis, J. (1988) Healed at last. *Nursing Times, Community Outlook* **84**: 32, August, 11–12.

Department of Health (1990) *Strategy for Nursing.* Department of Health, London.

Department of Health (1991) *The Patient's Charter.* HMSO, London.

Falanga, V. (1992) Growth factors and wound repair. *Journal of Tissue Viability* **2**: 3, 100–4.

Flanagan, M. (1992) Outside influences. *Nursing Times* **88**: 36, 72–78.

Gilchrist, B. (1989) Being accountable. *Nursing Times* **85**: 26, 67.

Green, J.W. & Wenzel, R.P. (1977) Post-operative wound infection. *Annals of Surgery* **185**, 264–8.

Greenhalgh, D.G., Sprugel, K.H., Murray, M.J. & Ross, R. (1990) PDGF and FGF stimulate wound healing in the genetically diabetic mouse. *American Journal of Pathology* **136**, 1235–46.

Gwyther, J. (1988) Skilled dressing. *Nursing Times* **84**: 19, 60–61.

Hibbs, P. (1988) *Pressure area care for the City & Hackney Health Authority.* City & Hackney Health Authority, London.

Johnson, A. (1985) The economics of modern wound management. *British Journal of Pharmaceutical Practice* **7**: 11, 294–6.

Lawrence, W.T., Norton, J.A., Sporn, M.B., Gorshboth, C. & Grotendorst, G.F. (1986) The reversal of an adriamycin induced healing impairment with chemoattractants and growth factors. *Annals of Surgery* **203**, 142–7.

Livesley, B. & Simpson, G. (1989) Hard cost of soft sores. *Health Service Journal* **99**: 5138, 231.

Milward, P. (1988) Personal Communication, Walsall Health Authority.

Ralph, C. (1990) Nursing management and leadership – the challenge. In Jolley, M. & Allan, P. (eds) *Current Issues in Nursing Development.* Croom Helm, Beckenham, Kent.

Royal College of Nursing (1990) *Accountability in Nursing – A Discussion Document.* RCN, London.

Robertson, J.C. (1984) Counting the cost. *Nursing Times* **83**: 39, 56.

Robson, M.C., Phillips, L.G., Thomason, A., Robson, L.E. & Pierce, G.F. (1992) Platelet-derived growth factor BB for the treatment of chronic pressure ulcers. *Lancet* **339**: 8784, 23–25.

Sporn, M.B. & Roberts, A.B. (1988) Peptide growth factors are multifunctional. *Nature* **332**, 217–19.

Sutton, J. & Wallace, A. (1990) Pressure sores: the views and practices of senior hospital doctors. *Care – Science and Practice* **8**: 3, 115–18.

Turner, T.D. (1992) Surgical dressings and their evolution. In Harding, K.G., Leaper, D.L. & Turner, T.D. (eds) *Proceedings of the 1st European Conference on Advances in Wound Management*. Macmillan Magazines Ltd., London.

Walsh, M. & Ford, P. (1989) *Nursing Rituals, Research and Rational Actions*. Heinemann Nursing, Oxford.

Wise, A. (1986) The social ulcer. *Nursing Times* **82**: 21, 47–49.

United Kingdom Central Council for Nursing, Midwifery and Health Visiting (1989) *Exercising Accountability*. UKCC, London.

United Kingdom Central Council for Nursing, Midwifery and Health Visiting (1992a) *The Code of Professional Conduct for the Nurse, Midwife and Health Visitor*. UKCC, London.

United Kingdom Central Council for Nursing, Midwifery and Health Visiting (1992b) *The Scope of Professional Practice*. UKCC, London.

United Kingdom Central Council for Nursing, Midwifery and Health Visiting (1993) *Standards for Records and Record Keeping*. UKCC, London.

Vaughan, B. (1989) Autonomy and accountability. *Nursing Times* **85**: 3, 54–55.

Appendix A
The Usage and Application of Proprietary Wound Management Products

PRODUCTS ACCORDING TO CATEGORY

ALGINATES

Fibracol, Kaltoclude, Kaltostat, Sorbsan, Tegagel.

ANTIBACTERIALS

Flammazine, Metrotop.

BEADS

Debrisan, Dermaproof, Iodoflex, Iodosorb.

CHARCOALS

Actisorb Plus, Carbonet, Clinflex Odour Control Dressing, Denidor, Kaltocarb, Lyofoam C.

FOAMS

Allevyn, Allevyn Cavity Wound, Lyofoam, Silastic Foam, Tielle.

HYDROCOLLOIDS

Biofilm, Comfeel, Cutinova hydro, Granuflex*, Tegasorb.

HYDROGELS

Bard Absorbtion Dressing, Gelliperm, Intrasite Gel, 2nd Skin, Vigilon.

LOW-ADHERENT (MEDICATED)

Inadine.

* Granuflex is known as Duoderm outside the UK

STREPTOKINASE/STREPTODORNASE

Varidase.

TULLES (NON-MEDICATED)

Mepitel.

VAPOUR-PERMEABLE FILMS

Bioclusive, Cutifilm, Dermoclude, Opraflex, Opsite Flexigrid, Tegaderm, Transite.

VAPOUR-PERMEABLE MEMBRANES

Omiderm, Spyroflex, Spyrosorb, Surfasoft, Tegapore.

PRODUCTS IN ALPHABETICAL ORDER

ACTISORB PLUS ™

Description

Activated charcoal with silver incorporated into a porous nylon sleeve.

Sizes

10.5 cm × 10.5 cm, 19 cm × 19.5 cm

Indications

Malodourous wounds, e.g. fungating carcinomas, leg ulcers or wounds contaminated with bacteria.

Contraindications

Patients sensitive to nylon.

How to apply

(1) Cleanse wound and dry skin around.
(2) Apply directly to wound or in conjunction with another product.

Supplementary dressings

Absorbent pad.
Tape or bandage.

How to remove

(1) Lift carefully from wound. Use saline to release if dressing has become adherent.

Frequency of dressing change

Daily initially, reducing to 3–7 days.
Frequency will vary if used in conjunction with other dressings.

Advantages

(1) Effective method of controlling odour.

Disadvantages

(1) Cannot be cut to size.
(2) May adhere to wound if used as a primary dressing.

ALLEVYN ™

Description

Polyurethane trilaminate structure with a non-adherent contact layer, absorbant foam central layer and waterproof outer layer.

Sizes

10 cm × 10 cm, 20 cm × 20 cm, 9 cm × 9 cm tracheostomy dressing.

Indications

Heavily exuding wounds, e.g. venous leg ulcers.

Contraindications

Known allergy to dressing.

How to apply

(1) Cleanse wound and dry skin around.
(2) Select size of dressing to allow a 2–3 cm margin around wound.
(3) Apply patterned side of dressing to wound.

Supplementary dressings

Tape or bandage.

How to remove

(1)   Loosen tape and lift dressing carefully from wound.

Frequency of dressing change

4–7 days depending on volume of exudate.

Advantages

(1)   Easy to apply.
(2)   Can be cut to shape/size of wound.

Disadvantages

(1)   May adhere if exudate becomes reduced.

ALLEVYN ™ CAVITY WOUND DRESSING

Description

Absorbant polyurethane foam chippings encased in a perforated film.

Sizes

5 cm circular; 10 cm circular; 9 cm × 2.5 cm tubular, 12 cm × 4 cm tubular.

Indications

All types of cavity wounds, e.g. surgical cavities or pressure sores.

Contraindications

Cavities filled with necrotic tissue.

How to apply

(1)   Cleanse wound and dry skin around.
(2)   Insert appropriate size/shape dressing into cavity.

Supplementary dressing

Absorbent pad or film dressing.
Tape.

How to remove

(1) Remove outer dressing.
(2) Gently remove dressing from cavity and discard.

Frequency of dressing change

1–5 days depending on degree of exudate.

Advantages

(1) Easy to apply.
(2) Highly absorbent.

Disadvantages

(1) Does not conform to cavity shape.
(2) The available sizes may be inappropriate for cavity size.

BARD ™ ABSORBTION DRESSING

Description

Flakes of a graft copolymer starch.

Sizes

3 g packet; 6 g packet.

Indications

Exuding sloughy or granulating wounds.

Contraindications

Necrotic wounds.
Patients with renal or cardiac impairment.

How to apply

(1) Cleanse wound and dry skin around.
(2) Using a sterile container mix flakes with sterile water (30 ml for 3 g; 60 ml for 6 g). Stir mixture. It will form a light brown slurry in 10–15 s.
(3) Using gloved finger, fill wound cavity to a depth of 1 cm. The dressing should not be tightly packed into the wound.

Supplementary dressing

Low-adherent dressing.
Absorbent pad.
Tape.

How to remove

(1) Remove outer dressing.
(2) Irrigate wound with normal saline.

Frequency of dressing change

1–2 days.

Advantages

(1) Deodorizes wound.
(2) Conformable to wound shape.

Disadvantages

(1) Expensive.
(2) Complicated dressing to use.

BIOCLUSIVE ™

Description

Vapour permeable polyurethane adhesive film.

Sizes

5.1 cm × 7.6 cm, 10.2 cm × 12.7 cm, 12.7 cm × 17.8 cm, 10.2 cm × 25.4 cm.

Indications

Superficial low-exuding wounds.
Grade 1 pressure sores.

Contraindications

Necrotic or infected wounds.
Cavity wounds.
Patients with thin, friable skin.

How to apply

(1)   Cleanse wound and dry skin around.
(2)   Apply protective skin wipe to intact skin.
(3)   Using an appropriate size to give a 2–4 cm margin around the wound, remove centre backing paper.
(4)   Position dressing over wound and remove side backing papers whilst smoothing onto skin.

Supplementary dressings

None.

How to remove

(1)   Lift two opposing edges and pull film laterally, allowing it to peel away from skin.

Frequency of dressing change

Up to 7 days.

Advantages

(1)   Dressing will pull apart if sticks to itself.
(2)   Wound can be monitored through dressing.
(3)   Patient may bath or shower.

Disadvantages

(1)   No absorptive capacity.

BIOFILM ®

Description

Adherent dressing consisting of polyisobutylene, sodium carboxymethylcellulose, pectin and gelatin with a non-woven semipermeable backing.

Sizes

10 cm × 10 cm; 20 cm × 20 cm; powder: 5 g sachet.

Indications

Wide range of moderate- to low-exuding wounds.

Contraindications

Infected wounds.
Grade IV pressure sores.

How to apply

(1) Cleanse wound and dry skin around.
(2) Select a size of dressing which will allow a 2–3 cm margin around the wound.
(3) Peel off backing paper and place over wound, smoothing into place.
(4) Biofilm powder may be used to fill small cavities before covering with the wafer.

Supplementary dressings

None.

How to remove

(1) Gently peel dressing away from wound.

NB As exudate is absorbed, the hydrocolloid forms a yellow gel. It has a distinctive odour which should not be mistaken for pus.

Frequency of dressing change

Up to 7 days, depending on the amount of exudate.
Criteria for change: wrinkling of dressing or leakage of exudate.

Advantages

(1) Easy to apply.
(2) Can be used on a wide range of wounds.

Disadvantages

(1) Does not have waterproof backing like other hydrocolloids.

CARBONET ™

Description

A three-layer dressing consisting of a low-adherent contact layer, an absorbent layer and an activated charcoal layer.

Sizes

10 cm × 10 cm, 10 cm × 20 cm.

Indications

Malodourous exuding wounds.

Contraindications

None known.

How to apply

(1) Cleanse wound and dry skin around.
(2) Apply shiny side of dressing to wound.

Supplementary dressings

Tape or bandages.

How to remove

(1) Loosen tape and lift dressing carefully from wound.

Frequency of dressing change

1–2 days depending on the amount of exudate.

Advantages

(1) Conformable, dressing can be cut to shape.

Disadvantages

(1) If little exudate, dressing may adhere to wound.

CLINIFLEX ODOUR CONTROL ™ DRESSING

Description

Activated charcoal cloth encased in viscose rayon.

Sizes

10 cm × 10 cm; 10 cm × 20 cm; 15 cm × 25 cm.

Indications

Secondary dressing for malodourous wounds.

Contraindications

None known.

How to apply

(1) Cleanse wound and dry skin around.
(2) Apply primary dressing to wound.
(3) Cover with Cliniflex.

Supplementary dressings

Tape or bandages.

How to remove

(1) Gently remove dressing from wound.

Frequency of dressing change

1–2 days depending on the amount of exudate.

Advantages

(1) Easy to use.
(2) Can be cut to size.

Disadvantages

(1) Not very absorbent.

COMFEEL ™

Description

Hydrocolloid dressing containing absorbent sodium carboxymethylcellulose, synthetic block-copolymer, tackifier resin and plasticizer as the adhesive mass. Available as wafer, paste and powder.

Sizes

4 cm × 6 cm; 10 cm × 10 cm; 15 cm × 15 cm; 20 cm × 20 cm, paste: 50 g; 12 g; powder: 6g
Comfeel Transparent ™: 5 cm × 7 cm, 9 cm × 14 cm; 15 cm × 20 cm.
Comfeel Extra Absorbent ™: 6 cm × 8.5 cm, 8.5 cm × 12 cm.

Indications

A wide range of wounds with moderate to low exudate.
Use Comfeel Transparent for superficial wounds.
Use Comfeel Extra Absorbent for more heavily exuding wounds.

Contraindications

Exposed muscle, tendon or bone.
Known allergy.
Use with caution on wounds caused by chronic infection such as tuberculosis or syphilis.
Under medical supervision on ischaemic diabetic ulcers.

How to apply

(1) Cleanse wound and dry skin around.
(2) Select a size of dressing to allow a margin of 1.5–2 cm around wound.
(3) Remove protective backing paper and apply dressing to wound.
(4) Paste or powder may be used under the wafer to fill small cavities.

Supplementary dressings

None.

How to remove

Gently peel dressing back from wound.
Irrigate wound to remove any residue.

Frequency of dressing change

Dressing may be left in place up to 7 days.
Criteria for dressing change: Comfeel becomes transparent over entire area or dressing leaks.

Advantages

(1) Easy to use.
(2) Waterproof, so patient may bathe or shower.
(3) Colour change indicates when to change dressing.

Disadvantages

(1) Unpleasant odour from gelled dressing at dressing change.

CUTIFILM ™

Description

A polyurethane adhesive film.

Sizes

5 cm × 7.5 cm; 7.5 cm × 10 cm; 10 cm × 14 cm.

Indications

Superficial, low exuding wounds.
Grade I pressure sores.

Contraindications

Infected wounds.
Heavily exuding wounds.

How to apply

(1) Cleanse wound and dry skin around.
(2) Apply protective skin wipe to intact skin.
(3) Using an appropriate size to allow a 2–3 cm margin around wound remove the two white release papers.
(4) Holding blue tabs, position dressing over wound and smooth in place.
(5) Use blue tab to remove backing from film.

Supplementary dressings

None.

How to remove

(1) Lift one edge and stretch lightly, allowing dressing to peel away.

Frequency of dressing change

Up to 7 days.

Advantages

(1) Wound may be monitored through dressing.
(2) Patient may bath or shower.

Disadvantages

(1)   No absorptive capacity.

CUTINOVA HYDRO ™

Description

A semi transparent polyurethane gel hydroactive dressing.

Sizes

6 cm × 5 cm; 10 cm × 10 cm; 20 cm × 15 cm.

Indications

Light to moderately exuding shallow wounds.

Contraindications

Do not use in direct contact with tendons or bones.
Infected wounds: use under medical supervision.

How to apply

(1)   Cleanse wound and dry skin around.
(2)   Select a suitable size of dressing to allow a 2 cm margin around wound.
(3)   Remove backing paper and apply dressing to wound.
(4)   Smooth dressing in place.

Supplementary dressings

None.

How to remove

(1)   Roll dressing back whilst applying light counter pressure to skin.

Frequency of dressing change

Up to 10 days.
Criteria for dressing change: whitish blister formed to the edge of the dressing.

Advantages

(1)   Unlike other hydrocolloids this dressing does not gel.

(2) Wound can be partially observed through dressing.
(3) Waterproof so patient can bath or shower.

Disadvantages

(1) Cannot be used on such a wide range of wounds as other hydrocolloids.

DEBRISAN ™

Description

Hydrophilic beads made from dextranomer either combined as a paste or in textile bags.

Sizes

Paste: 10 g; Pads: 6 cm × 4 cm.

Indications

Moderate to heavily exuding necrotic, infected or sloughy wounds.

Contraindications

Low exuding wounds.
Granulating wounds.
Narrow sinuses where removal may be difficult.

How to apply

(1) Cleanse wound and dry skin around.
(2) Open gauze piece to single thickness and lay over wound.
(3) Spread paste to depth of at least 0.6 cm over gauze, to cover wound area.
(4) Fold excess gauze over paste.
(5) If using pads: place pads in wound, they need not cover entire wound surface.

Supplementary dressings

Absorbent pads.
Wide tape or strapping.

How to remove

(1) Gently remove strapping and old dressing.
(2) Irrigate wound with saline if dressing adheres.

Frequency of dressing change

Twice daily-2 days, depending on the degree of exudate.

Advantages

(1) Useful in the early stages of wound debridement.

Disadvantages

(1) Expensive.

DENIDOR ™

Description

Activated charcoal pad.

Sizes

17.5 cm × 19 cm.

Indications

Malodourous wounds.

Contraindications

None known.

How to apply

(1) This dressing is not sterile, so should not be placed in contact with the wound.
(2) Apply suitable primary dressing.
(3) Cover with low-adherent dressing.
(4) Apply Denidor.

Supplementary dressings

Absorbent pad.
Tape or bandage.

How to remove

(1) Lift carefully from wound. Use saline to release if dressing has become adherent.

Frequency of dressing change

Daily.

Advantages

(1)   Assists in controlling odour.

Disadvantages

(1)   Not sterile.
(2)   Cannot be cut to size.

DERMAPROOF ®

Description

Granules of mucopolysaccharides contained within a non-woven polypropylene mesh sachet.

Sizes

4 cm × 4 cm sachet or pad.

Indications

Infected or sloughy exuding wounds.

Contraindications

Hard necrotic eschar.
Low exuding wounds.
Granulating and epithelializing wounds.

How to apply

(1)   Cleanse wound and dry skin around.
(2)   Apply pad to wound.

Supplementary dressings

Absorbent pads.
Bandage or tape.

How to remove

(1)   Loosen and remove outer dressings.
(2)   Gently lift pad from wound.

Frequency of dressing change

1–4 days depending on the amount of exudate.

Advantages

(1) Easy to use.

Disadvantages

(1) Expensive.

DERMOCLUDE ™

Description

Vapour-permeable film made of a light copolymer film.

Sizes

10 cm × 10 cm; 15 cm × 20 cm.

Indications

Superficial clean wounds with low to no exudate.

Contraindications

Infected wounds.
Wounds with heavy exudate.
When there is fragile skin around wound.

How to apply

(1) Cleanse wound and dry skin around.
(2) Apply protective skin wipe to intact skin.
(3) Remove backing film from adhesive surface.
(4) Apply dressing to wound.
(5) Remove transparent carrier by gently lifting white tab.
(6) Smooth dressing in place.

Supplementary dressings

None.

How to remove

(1) Gently lift the corner of the dressing and peel back from wound.

Frequency of dressing change

1–7 days.
Criteria for dressing change: leakage of exudate, wrinkling or slipping of dressing.

Advantages

(1) Allows wound to be seen through dressing.

Disadvantages

(1) No absorptive capacity.

FIBRACOL ™

Description

Fibracol is a combination of 90% collagen and 10% calcium alginate in a flat pad.

Sizes

9.5 cm × 9.5 cm.

Indications

Moderate to heavily exuding wounds.

Contraindications

Wounds with low to no exudate.

How to apply

(1) Cleanse wound and dry skin around.
(2) Position Fibracol over wound.

Supplementary dressings

Absorbent pads.
Bandage or tape.

How to remove

(1) Loosen and remove outer dressings.
(2) Gently lift dressing from wound.

Frequency of dressing change

1–7 days depending on the amount of exudate.

Advantages

(1) Easy to use.
(2) May be cut to size.
(3) Maintains integrity when wet.

Disadvantages

(1) Only available in one size.

FLAMMAZINE ™

Description

A hydrophilic cream containing silver sulphadiazine 1% w/w.

Sizes

50 g tube.

Indications

Burns.
Effective against *Pseudomonas* and *Staphylococcus aureus*

Contraindications

Impairment of renal or hepatic function.
Sensitivity may occur, but uncommon.
Heavily exudating ulcers.

How to apply

(1) Clean wound with saline, dry skin around.
(2) Apply cream to wound with finger using sterile glove.
(3) Take care not to spread cream onto surrounding skin as will cause maceration.

NB Burns require specialist management

Supplementary dressings

Low adherent dressings.
Absorbent pad.
Tape or bandage.

How to remove

(1)   Irrigate wound with saline.

Frequency of dressing change

At least once daily.

Advantages

(1)   Effective anti-bacterial cream.

Disadvantages

(1)   May cause skin maceration.
(2)   Relatively expensive.
(3)   When used on infected wounds, need to change to a different dressing when infection cleared.

GELLIPERM ™

Description

A hydrogel containing polyacrylamide, agar and 96% water.

Sizes

Gelliperm Wet: 26 cm × 12 cm; 13 cm × 12 cm; Gelliperm Dry 25 cm × 11 cm; Gelliperm Granulate: 20 g and 50 g tubes.

Indications

A wide range of wounds with moderate to low exudate.

Contraindications

Wounds with a necrotic eschar.
Wounds infected with *Pseudomonas sp*.
Cavities where the extent of the wound is not known.

How to apply

(1)   Cleanse wound and dry skin around.
(2)   Gelliperm Wet: apply a suitable size to cover wound, an overlap is unnecessary.
(3)   Gelliperm Granulate: fill wound with Gelliperm granules.

Supplementary dressings

Absorbent pads.
Strapping or tape.

How to remove

(1) Gently remove strapping and old dressing.
(2) Irrigate wound with saline to remove any remaining dressing.

Frequency of dressing change

Every 1–3 days.
Gelliperm Wet can be rehydrated with saline daily. A strict aseptic technique should be used.

Advantages

(1) Easy to remove.

Disadvantages

(1) Relatively expensive.
(2) Dehydrates very quickly, rehydration is messy.

GRANUFLEX ™ (Improved Formulation)

Description

Granuflex consists of an outer layer of waterproof polyurethane foam bonded to a matrix of hydrocolloid particles (gelatin, pectin and methylcellulose) and a hydrophobic polymer.
NB Improved Formulation Granuflex is referred to as Granuflex in this text.

Sizes

10 cm × 10 cm; 15 cm × 20 cm; 20 cm × 20 cm; 20 cm × 30 cm, Paste: 30 g tube;
Granuflex Extra Thin: 7.5 cm × 7.5 cm; 10 cm × 10 cm; 15 cm × 15 cm;
Granuflex Bordered: 6 cm × 6 cm; 10 cm × 10 cm, 15 cm × 15 cm; 10 cm × 13 cm; 15 cm × 18 cm.

Indications

A wide range of wounds to a depth of 4–5 cm.
Granuflex paste for shallow cavities.

Granuflex Extra Thin for for lightly exuding wounds, especially where flexibility is needed.
Granuflex for moderate to heavily exuding wounds.
Granulex Bordered for more awkward areas such as the sacrum.

Contraindications

Immunosupressed patients, e.g. leukaemia.
Wounds with exposed tendon or bone: Granuflex should only be used under medical supervision.
Ulcers resulting from infections such as tuberculosis, syphillis and deeper fungal infections.
Full-thickness burns greater than 2% body surface area.

How to apply

(1) Select a suitable type and size of Granuflex.
(2) Cleanse wound and dry skin around.
(3) Ensure that the dressing is large enough to ensure an overlap of 2–3 cm beyond wound margin. When cutting larger wafers to size, curve corners.
(4) Remove backing paper and apply wafer to wound in a rolling motion.
(5) Smooth in place, particularly around edges. Adhesion improves as the dressing warms.
(6) Fill small cavities with paste before applying wafer.

Supplementary dressings

None.

How to remove

(1) Gently peel dressing away from skin. Free edges of dressing all around before lifting from wound.
(2) It may be helpful to use a sterile paper towel to prevent any dribbles of gel running from wound.

NB As the dressing absorbs exudate, the hydrocolloid layer liquifies into a gel. This looks like pus and has a distinctive odour. This is normal, but patients should be told so in advance.

Frequency of dressing change

Every 3–7 days, depending on the amount of exudate.
Criteria for change: leakage of exudate or wrinkling or sliding of dressing.

Advantages

(1)   Easy to use.
(2)   Waterproof so patient can bath or shower.

Disadvantages

(1)   Odour very offensive to some.
(2)   Hydrocolloid layer may squeeze out of sides of wafer if applied to weight bearing areas.

INADINE ™

Description

Rayon dressing impregnated with 10% povidone iodine absorbent ointment.

Sizes

5 cm × 5 cm; 9.5 cm × 9.5 cm.

Indications

Shallow infected wounds.
Contaminated traumatic injuries.
Superficial burns.

Contraindications

(1)   Known allergy to povidone iodine or iodine.
(2)   Heavily exuding wounds.

How to apply

(1)   Clean wound with saline and dry skin around.
(2)   Apply Inadine dressing to cover wound. Up to 4 pieces of Inadine may be used to cover the surface area of a large wound. In the case of babies, not more than 10% of body surface area should be covered.

Supplementary dressings

Absorbent pad.
Tape or bandage.

How to remove

Gently peel back from wound and remove.

Frequency of dressing change

Criteria for dressing change: when Inadine becomes white.
1–7 days depending on exudate.
If using more than 3 pieces, dressing should not be used for more than 4 days without seeking medical opinion.

Advantages

(1) Broad-spectrum antiseptic effect.
(2) Easy to use.
(3) No reports of acquired resistance.

Disadvantages

(1) Little absorptive capacity.
(2) Should not be used for more than a period of 3–4 weeks.

INTRASITE GEL ™

Description

A hydrogel containing a Graft-T-Starch copolymer.

Sizes

15 g, 25 g sachets.

Indications

Necrotic tissue.
Sloughy deep or shallow wounds.
Granulating deep or shallow wounds.
Epithelializing wounds.
Sinuses.

Contraindications

Should not be used with iodine preparations.

How to apply

(1) Cleanse wound and dry skin around.
(2) Intrasite Gel may be squeezed directly into the wound or onto a low-adherent dressing, whichever is easier.
(3) It should be applied to a depth of 1 cm on necrotic tissue and 0.5 cm on other wounds.
(4) Apply via a syringe and filling cannula into sinuses.

Supplementary dressings

Low-adherent dressings.
Absorbent pad.
Tape or bandage.

How to remove

(1) Gently remove secondary dressings.
(2) Irrigate wound with saline.

Frequency of dressing change

Daily in the presence of necrotic tissue. Every 1–3 days depending on the volume of exudate.

Advantages

(1) Easy to apply.
(2) Cost-effective.
(3) Reduces wound pain.
(4) Versatile in use.

Disadvantages

(1) There may be wastage as whatever remains in the sachet must be discarded.
(2) If the incorrect depth of dressing is used, the wound may dry out around the edges.

IODOFLEX ™

Description

Units of cadexomer iodine paste.

Size

5 g.

Indications

Heavily exuding sloughy, infected or necrotic chronic wounds, especally leg ulcers.

Contraindications

Known or suspected iodine sensitivity.
Hashimoto's thyroiditis.

History of Grave's disease.
Non-toxic nodular goitre.
Pregnant or lactating women.
When the following drugs are being taken: lithium, sulphafurazoles, sulphonylureas.

How to apply

(1) Cleanse wound and dry skin around.
(2) Remove the carrier gauze on both sides of the dressing and apply to the wound.
(3) More than one dressing may be required to cover the wound. No more than 10 dressings (50 g) should be used each time.

Supplementary dressings

Absorbent pads.
Tape or bandage.

How to remove

(1) Gently lift dressing from wound. Soak dressing with saline if it has become adherent.
(2) Cleanse any remaining Iodoflex away with saline.

Frequency of dressing change

3 times weekly.

Advantages

(1) Easy to apply.
(2) Highly absorbant.

Disadvantages

(1) Expensive.
(2) A course of treatment should not last more than three months.

IODOSORB ™

Description

A cadexomer preparation in the form of powder or ointment.

Sizes

Powder: 3 g sachets; Ointment: 10 g tubes.

Indications

Necrotic, infected or sloughy chronic wounds with moderate to heavy exudate.

Contraindications

Known or suspected iodine sensitivity.
Hashimoto's thyroiditis.
History of Grave's disease.
Non-toxic nodular goitre.
Patients taking lithium, sulphafurazoles or sulphonylureas.
Pregnant or lactating women.

How to apply

(1) Cleanse wound and dry skin around.
(2) Apply powder or ointment to wound to a depth of 3 mm. No more than 16 sachets or 5 tubes should be used in any one application.

Supplementary dressings

Absorbent pad.
Strapping or tape.

How to remove

(1) Gently remove outer dressings.
(2) Remove remnants of dressing by irrigating wound with saline.

Frequency of dressing change

Every 1–3 days depending on the amount of exudate.
Criteria for change: loss of colour of powder or ointment.

Advantages

(1) Iodine is a broad-spectrum antiseptic.

Disadvantages

(1) Relatively expensive.
(2) No more than 150 g should be applied in a week.
(3) Course of treatment should not exceed 3 months.

KALTOCARB ™

Description

Consists of three layers: an alginate wound contact layer bonded to an activated charcoal layer, bonded to an outer layer of polyester and viscose.

Sizes

7.5 cm × 12 cm.

Indications

Moderate to heavily exuding malodourous wounds.

Contraindications

Wounds with little or no exudate.

How to apply

(1) Cleanse wound and dry skin around.
(2) Apply dressing to wound.

Supplementary dressings

Absorbent pads.
Tape or bandage.

How to remove

Loosen outer dressings and gently remove from wound.
Frequency of dressing change
Every 1–2 days depending on the amount of exudate.

Advantages

(1) Combines the benefit of an alginate with odour control.
(2) Easy to use.

Disadvantages

(1) Only one size available.

KALTOCLUDE ™

Description

A vapour-permeable film combined with a smaller alginate (Kaltostat ™) pad.

Sizes

10 cm × 10 cm; 15 cm × 20 cm.

Indications

Superficial low exuding wounds.

Contraindications

Wounds with no exudate, especially those with a necrotic eschar.

How to apply

(1) Clean wound and dry skin around.
(2) Remove backing sheet from adhesive surface and apply dressing to wound.
(3) Remove transparent film carrier from dressing by gently pulling white tab.
(4) Smooth dressing in place.

Supplementary dressings

None.

How to remove

(1) Gently lift one corner of the film and peel back.

Frequency of dressing change

3–7 days depending on exudate.

Advantages

(1) Simple to use.
(2) Infrequent dressing change.

Disadvantages

(1) Care is needed to prevent the film damaging fragile skin.

KALTOSTAT ⓉⓂ

Description

A fibrous dressing containing 80% calcium alginate and 20% sodium alginate.

Sizes

5 cm × 5 cm; 7.5 cm × 12 cm; 10 cm × 20 cm; 15 cm × 25 cm; 30 cm × 60 cm; Packing: 2 g, Kaltostat Fortex ® 10 cm × 10 cm.

Indications

Management of bleeding wounds.
A range of moderate to heavily exuding wounds.
Kaltostat Packing for cavity wounds.
Kaltostat Fortex for excessively exuding wounds.

Contraindications

Low exuding wounds.
Wounds with a dry necrotic eschar.

How to apply

(1)   Cleanse wound and dry skin around.
(2)   Select a suitable size dressing to cover wound.
(3)   If using Packing, fill cavity loosely.

Supplementary dressings

Absorbent pad.
Tape or bandage.

How to remove

(1)   Loosen outer dressings and remove.
(2)   If Kaltostat has become adherent, irrigate back of dressing with saline and remove.

Frequency of dressing change

Infected wounds should be changed daily.
Other wounds, every 2–7 days depending on the amount of exudate.

Advantages

(1)   Easy to use.

Disadvantages

(1)   Will adhere to wound if there is insufficient exudate.

LYOFOAM ®

Description

A polyurethane foam sheet, the wound contact side is smooth and hydrophilic, the backing layer is hydrophobic.
Lyofoam A has a waterproof, adhesive foam backing.

Sizes

7.5 cm × 7.5 cm; 10 cm × 10 cm; 17.5 cm × 10 cm; 25 cm × 10 cm; 20 cm × 15 cm; 30 cm × 25 cm; 70 cm × 40 cm.
Lyofoam A: 10 cm × 10 cm.

Indications

Granulating or epithelializing shallow wounds with low to moderate exudate.
Lyofoam A may be used on sacral sores in incontinent patients.

Contraindications

Wounds covered with a dry eschar.
Wounds with no exudate.

How to apply

(1)   Cleanse wound and dry skin around.
(2)   Select a size of dressing which will allow a 2–3 cm margin around the wound.
(3)   Apply shiny side of dressing to wound.
(4)   Lyofoam A must have backing paper removed.

Supplementary dressings

Adhesive tapes. None for Lyofoam A.

How to remove

(1)   Loosen tapes along the edge of the dressing.
(2)   Gently lift dressing from wound.

Frequency of dressing change

1–7 days depending on the amount of exudate.
Criteria for dressing change: exudate leaking along edge of dressing.

Advantages

(1) Easy to use.
(2) Conformable.
(3) Stays in position over awkward areas.

Disadvantages

(1) Will adhere to wound if there is no exudate.

LYOFOAM C ™

Description

Lyofoam dressing with an activated charcoal layer adhered to the back of the dressing and sealed to it with a thin layer of polyurethane.

Sizes

10 cm × 10 cm; 20 cm × 15 cm; 25 cm × 10 cm.

Indications

Malodourous wounds with low to moderate exudate.

Contraindications

Wounds with a dry eschar.

How to apply

(1) Cleanse wound and dry skin around.
(2) Select a suitable size dressing to allow a 2–3 cm margin around wound.
(3) Apply shiny side of dressing to wound.

Supplementary dressings

Tape or bandage.

How to remove

(1) Loosen tapes around the dressing edge.
(2) Gently lift dressing from the wound.

Frequency of dressing change

1–4 days depending on the amount of exudate.

Advantages

(1) Simple to use.
(2) An effective combination of dressing and charcoal.

Disadvantages

(1) Absorbs less exudate than ordinary Lyofoam.

MEPITEL ™

Description

A fine mesh polyamide netting enclosed in silicone gel.

Sizes

5 cm × 7.5 cm; 7.5 cm × 10 cm; 10 cm × 18 cm; 20 cm × 30 cm.

Indications

Over skin grafts.
Superficial wounds.

Contraindications

Heavily exuding wounds.
Necrotic, sloughy or infected wounds.

How to apply

(1) Cleanse wound and dry skin around.
(2) Select a suitable size to allow a 2 cm margin around wound.
(3) Remove backing paper and apply to wound.

Supplementary dressings

Absorbent pad.
Tape or bandage.

How to remove

Lift gently from wound.

Frequency of dressing change

3–4 days.
NB outer pad can be changed leaving Mepitel in place.

Advantages

(1) Adheres to surrounding skin without adhering to wound.

Disadvantages

(1) Requires a margin of healthy skin around wound.
(2) Can only be applied to flat or convex areas. Cannot be applied to concave areas, e.g. neck or groin.

METROTOP ™

Description

Colourless gel containing metronidazole BP 0.8%.

Size

30 g tube.

Indications

Malodourous fungating tumours.
Malodourous wounds when other methods have failed.

Contraindications

Known hypersensitivity to metronidazole.
Pregnancy or lactation.

How to apply

(1) Cleanse wound and dry skin around.
(2) Apply protective skin wipe to fragile or sore intact skin around wound.
(3) Apply Metrotop thickly to wound.
NB Metrotop may be combined with Intrasite Gel ™ to give a thicker consistency, but this does dilute the strength of the Metrotop.

Supplementary dressings

Low adherent dressing.
Absorbent pad.
Tape or bandage.

How to remove

(1) Lift outer dressing carefully from wound. Use saline to release if dressing has become adherent.

Frequency of dressing change

Daily.

Advantages

(1)   An effective method of controlling odour by being active against the anaerobic bacteria which are responsible.

Disadvantages

(1)   No absorptive capacity.
(2)   Outer dressings may become adherent if dressing applied incorrectly.

OMIDERM ™

Description

A non-adhesive membrane of polyurethane bonded with hydrophilic monomers.

Sizes

5 cm × 7 cm; 8 cm × 10 cm; 18 cm × 10 cm; 60 cm × 10 cm; 21 cm × 31 cm.

Indications

Superficial and partial-thickness burns.
Surgical dermabrasions.
Skin donor sites (once haemostasis achieved).
Grazes and minor abrasions.
Radiation burns.
Other superficial wounds.

Contraindications

Known sensitivity to polyurethane.
Infected, bleeding or heavily exuding wounds.
Full-thickness wounds.

How to apply

(1)   Cleanse wound and dry skin around.
(2)   Select a suitable size dressing to allow a 1–2 cm margin beyon the wound.
(3)   Apply dressing onto wound without stretching it.
(4)   Carefully smooth dressing in place from the centre, thus removing all air bubbles and wrinkles. (This is most easily done wearing gloves.)
(5)   Check for good adherence to surrounding skin.

Supplementary dressings

Low-adherent dressing.
Absorbent pad.
Bandage or tape.

How to remove

(1) Loosen and remove outer dressings.
(2) Soak Omiderm with saline and gently remove.

Frequency of dressing change

Dressing change is usually unnecessary until wound is healed or the dressing peels off.
    The dressing should be changed if there are indications of infection or haematoma.
    The outer dressings should be changed to allow regular inspection of the wound.
    As wound heals and reduces in size, the dressing will peel off the healed area. Omiderm should be trimmed to maintain a 1 cm border around wound.

Advantages

(1) Highly vapour permeable.
(2) Infrequent dressing change.

Disadvantages

(1) A little complicated to use.

OPRAFLEX ™

Description

A polyurethane adhesive film dressing.

Sizes

5 cm × 7 cm; 10 cm × 12 cm; 10 cm × 25 cm; 15 cm × 20 cm; 30 cm × 20 cm.

Indications

Superficial granulating or epithelializing wounds with low to no exudate.
Postoperative surgical wounds.
Over bony prominences to prevent friction leading to pressure sores.

Contraindications

Wounds with moderate or greater exudate.
Infected wounds.

How to apply

(1)   Cleanse wound and dry skin around.
(2)   Wipe protective skin wipe over intact skin.
(3)   Select an appropriate size to allow a 2–3 cm margin around wound.
(4)   Bend back dressing to release the orange 'crackback' opening.
(5)   Peel off the cover paper from the 'crackback' one side at a time.
(6)   Holding the handles apply the dressing to the wound with the shiny side uppermost.
(7)   Pull at one handle to remove applicator and smooth dressing in place.

Supplementary dressings

None.

How to remove

Gently peel dressing from wound.

Frequency of dressing change

1–7 days depending on the amount of exudate.

Advantages

(1)   Easy to observe wound through dressing.

Disadvantages

(1)   No absorptive capacity.

OPSITE FLEXIGRID ™

Description

An adhesive polyurethane film dressing.

Sizes

10 cm × 12 cm; 15 cm × 20 cm; 12 cm × 25 cm.

Indications

Superficial clean wounds with no to low exudate.
Postoperative wounds.
Grade I pressure sores.
In conjunction with Intrasite Gel ™ or Varidase ™ over necrotic eschar.

Contraindications

Moderate to heavily exuding wounds.
Infected wounds.
Patients with thin friable intact skin.

How to apply

(1)   Cleanse wound and dry skin around.
(2)   Wipe protective skin wipe over intact skin.
(3)   Select a suitable size to allow a 3 cm margin around wound.
(4)   Peel off backing paper and apply dressing to wound.
(5)   If wished, a tracing of the wound outline can be made on the Flexigrid carrier. The carrier can then be removed from the outer side of the dressing.

NB: When applying over joints, maintain full flexion during application. Opsite Flexigrid may be cut and applied in strips.

Supplementary dressings

None.

How to remove

(1)   Gently lift a corner of the dressing from the wound.
(2)   Stretch the dressing parallel with the skin whilst holding the dressing down.
(3)   Repeat until all the dressing is removed.

NB stretching the dressing in this way breaks the adhesive and allows removal without trauma.

Frequency of dressing change

Up to 7 days.
Criteria for dressing change: leakage of exudate, wrinkling of dressing, obvious signs of wound infection.

Advantages

(1)   Allows observation of the wound through the dressing.

(2) Conformable.
(3) Allows easy mapping of the wound.
(4) Easy to apply.
(5) Cheap.

Disadvantages

(1) No absorptive capacity.

2ND SKIN ⓉⓂ

Description

A transparent hydrogel sheet made of 96% water and 4% polyethylene oxide.

Sizes

5 cm × 7.5 cm; 7.5 cm × 10 cm.

Indications

Superficial wounds with moderate to low exudate.

Contraindications

Wounds with necrotic eschar.
Infected wounds.
Heavily exuding wounds.

How to apply

(1) Cleanse wound and dry skin around.
(2) Remove blue polythene film and apply exposed side of dressing to wound.
(3) The remaining clear film may left *in situ* or removed (if left in place this provides an occlusive mode).

Supplementary dressings

Absorbent pad.
Bandage or tape.

How to remove

(1) Loosen and remove outer dressing.
(2) If dressing has become dehydrated, irrigate with saline before gently removing from wound.

Frequency of dressing change

1–3 days depending on the amount of exudate.

Advantages

Soothing cool feeling to wound.

Disadvantages

(1) Dehydrates quickly.
(2) Relatively expensive.

SILASTIC FOAM ™

Description

A two component dressing consisting of a silicone base and a catalyst which, when mixed, form a spongy elastomer.

Sizes

20 ml; 500 g pots.

Indications

Deep cavity granulating wounds.
Broad excision surgical wounds.

Contraindications

Infected wounds.
Cavity wounds with sinus formation.

How to apply

(1) Cleanse wound and dry skin around.
(2) Use plastic spatula to thoroughly mix silicone base in white plastic pot.
(3) Pour catalyst into plastic pot. Replace cap on catalyst tube.
(4) Stir mixture thoroughly for 15 seconds.
(5) Pour mixture into wound. It is very runny at this stage and it may be necessary to scoop the mixture back into the wound with the spatula.
(6) After 3 minutes the mixture will have set to a spongy foam four times its original size. Lift from wound to loosen and then replace.

Supplementary dressings

Absorbent pad.
Tape.

Daily routine

(1) This procedure should be carried out twice daily.
(2) Wearing plastic gloves, remove foam from wound and rinse under tap, squeezing gently.
(3) Place foam stent in a disposable receiver and soak in chlorhexidine 0.05% in 70% IMS for 10 minutes.
(4) Rinse stent under tap, squeeze gently and dry with paper towels.
(5) Replace in wound.

Frequency of dressing change

It is generally necessary to make a new stent weekly as the wound decreases in size.

Advantages

(1) Conforms to the shape of the wound.
(2) Excellent alternative to ribbon gauze packing.
(3) Easily removed without trauma to wound.

Disadvantages

(1) Requires skill to mix and mould.

SORBSAN ™

Description

A dressing consisting of calcium salt of alginic acid derived from seaweed.

Sizes

Flat dressing: 5 cm × 5 cm; 10 cm × 10 cm; 10 cm × 20 cm.
Sorbsan + ™ (incorporates a viscose pad): 7.5 cm × 10 cm; 10 cm × 15 cm.
Sorbsan SA ™ (with adhesive foam backing): 5 cm × 7 cm; 9 cm × 11 cm.
Sorbsan Packing ™: 30 cm long.
Sorbsan Ribbon ™: 40 cm long.

Indications

Any wound with moderate to heavy exudate.
Sorbsan + for shallow wounds with heavy exudate.

Sorbsan SA for small wounds with moderate exudate, especially in awkward areas. Not suitable for infected wounds.
Sorbsan Packing or Ribbon for cavity wounds.

Contraindications

Wounds with little exudate.

How to apply

(1) Cleanse wound and dry skin around.
(2) Select a suitable type and size of Sorbsan.
(3) Apply dressing to wound, if using Packing or Ribbon insert loosely into the cavity.

Supplementary dressings

Absorbent pad.
Bandage or tape.
None required for Sorbsan SA.

How to remove

(1) Loosen and remove outer dressings.
(2) Gently lift Sorbsan from wound.
(3) Irrigate any remaining fibres with saline to remove.

Frequency of dressing change

Daily for infected wounds.
1–4 days depending on amount of exudate.

Advantages

(1) Easy to use.
(2) Packing and Ribbon are an excellent alternative to ribbon gauze.

Disadvantages

(1) Once there is little exudate need to use a different dressing.
(2) Sometimes difficult to remove all crust around the wound margins.

SPYROFLEX ™

Description

A vapour permeable dressing consisting of an absorbent polyurethane membrane and a hydrophilic acrylic adhesive.

Sizes

10 cm × 10 cm; 20 cm × 20 cm.

Indications

Abrasions and lacerations.
An alternative to skin sutures.
Wounds over difficult contours of the body.

Contraindications

Infected wounds.
Wounds with moderate to heavy exudate.

How to apply

(1)   Cleanse wound and dry skin around.
(2)   Peel backing paper from dressing and apply to wound.
(3)   Over awkward areas, such as the hand, the dressing may be cut to shape.

Supplementary dressings

None.

How to remove

(1)   Lift a corner of the dressing and gently peel from wound.

Frequency of dressing change

1–7 days.

Advantages

(1)   Conforms to difficult contours.
(2)   Good adherence.

Disadvantages

(1)   Little absorptive capacity.

SPYROSORB ®

Description

A vapour-permeable dressing with three layers: an outer moisture responsive semipermeable polyurethane film; an absorbant polyurethane membrane, and a pressure-sensitive hydrophilic acrylic adhesive.

Sizes

10 cm × 10 cm; 20 cm × 20 cm.

Indications

Light to moderately exuding wounds.
Wounds over awkward contours of the body.

Contraindications

Infected wounds.

How to apply

(1) Cleanse wound and dry skin around.
(2) Peel off backing paper and apply dressing to wound allowing a 3 cm margin.
(3) Dressing may be cut to fit around awkward areas.

Supplementary dressings

None.

How to remove

(1) Lift corner of dressing and gently peel back from wound.

Frequency of dressing change

Up to 7 days.
Criteria for dressing change: when absorbed exudate is seen within 2 cm of the edge of the dressing.

Advantages

(1) Conforms to difficult contours.
(2) Good adherence.

Disadvantages

(1) Will not absorb heavy exudate.

SURFASORT ™

Description

Mesh made from monofilament woven polyamide thread.

Sizes

20 cm × 33 cm.

Indications

Skin graft fixation.

Contraindictions

None known.

How to apply

(1)   Immerse Surfasoft in saline for a few seconds.
(2)   Apply over skin graft to ensure good contact. The sheet may be cut if required.
(3)   Anchor Surfasoft with staples or sutures.
(4)   Excessive blood or fluid may be wiped from surface.

Supplementary dressings

A layer of damp gauze or non-woven material.
Absorbent pad.
Bandage.

How to remove

(1)   Remove outer dressings.
(2)   Soak Surfasoft in saline before gently lifting from wound.

Frequency of dressing change

Outer dressings should be changed daily.
Staples or sutures may be removed at 5 days.
Surfasoft can be removed after 7–14 days.

Advantages

(1)   Does not cause trauma to wound on removal.
(2)   Can be used on difficult anatomical areas, such as neck or groin.

Disadvantages

(1)   Removal of staples or sutures requires analgesia.

TEGADERM ®

Description

A thin polyurethane film coated with acrylic adhesive.

Sizes

6 cm × 7 cm; 10 cm × 12 cm; 10 cm × 25 cm; 15 cm × 20 cm; 20 cm × 30 cm.

Indications

Low to no exuding wounds.
Grade I pressure sores.
Surgically closed wounds and minor abrasions.

Contraindications

Infected wounds.
Necrotic eschar.
Wounds with moderate to heavy exudate.

How to apply

(1) Cleanse wound and dry skin around.
(2) Wipe protective skin wipe over intact skin.
(3) Select a suitable size to allow a 2–3 cm margin around the wound.
(4) Separate the centre cut-out on the dressing from the frame and discard.
(5) Remove the printed liner to reveal the wound contact side of the dressing.
(6) Holding the frame around the dressing, position it and smooth in place.
(7) Peel off the frame from and around the film and smooth the edges.

Supplementary dressings

None.

How to remove

(1) Gently lift one corner of the dressing and pull back towards the centre of the wound.

Frequency of dressing change

Up to 7 days.
Criteria for dressing change: leakage of exudate, wrinkling or slipping of dressing.

Advantages

(1) Easy to apply.
(2) Wound clearly visible through the dressing.

Disadvantages

(1) No absorptive capacity.

TEGAGEL ™

Description

A non-woven dressing made from fibres of calcium alginate.

Sizes

5 cm × 5 cm; 10 cm × 10 cm

Indications

Moderate to heavily exuding shallow wounds.

Contraindications

Caution with infected wounds.
Cavity wounds.

How to apply

(1) Cleanse wound and dry skin around.
(2) Select a suitable size to allow a small overlap onto the surrounding skin.
(3) Apply dressing to wound.

Supplementary dressings

Absorbent pad.
Bandage or tape.

How to remove

(1) Loosen and remove outer dressings.
(2) Gently lift Tegagel from wound.
(3) Soak dressing with saline if it has become adherent.

Frequency of dressing change

1–7 days depending on the amount of exudate.

Advantages

(1) Easy to use.

Disadvantages

(1) May become adherent to wound.

TEGAPORE ™

Description

A wound contact material made of hypoallergenic polyamide.

Sizes

7.5 cm × 10 cm; 7.5 cm × 20 cm; 20 cm × 25 cm.

Indications

Delicate exuding wounds.

Contraindications

None known.

How to apply

(1) Cleanse wound and dry skin around.
(2) Apply protective skin wipe to delicate intact skin.
(3) Tegapore may be applied wet or dry, depending on exudate.
(4) Apply to wound with a 5 mm border aound edge of wound.

Supplementary dressings

Absorbent pad.
Bandage or tape.

How to remove

(1) If wound surface is dry, moisten before removal.

Frequency of dressing change

Up to 14 days.
Outer dressings should be changed more frequently.

Advantages

(1) Wound can be observed through dressing.
(2) Dressing will not adhere to wound.

Disadvantages

(1) Need to become accustomed to wound appearance through dressing.

TEGASORB ®

Description

The dressing consists of a hydrocolloid adhesive covered with an outer clear adhesive film which extends beyond the hydrocolloid mass.

Sizes

Ovals: 7 cm × 9 cm; 10 cm × 12 cm; 14 cm × 17 cm.

Indications

Shallow wounds with moderate to low exudate.

Contraindications

Infected wounds.
Wounds involving muscle, tendon or bone.
Ulcers resulting from infections such as tuberculosis, syphilis and deep systemic fungal infections.
Wounds in patients with active vasculitis.

How to apply

(1) Cleanse wound and dry skin around.
(2) Select a suitable size to allow a 2–3 cm margin around the wound.
(3) Remove paper liner by lifting and pulling the red square end tab marked '1'.
(4) Apply adhesive side of dressing to wound and smooth film edges in place.
(5) Peel off delivery film by lifting and pulling white tabs marked '2'.
(6) Tear off red square end tab along perforations.

Supplementary dressings

None.

How to remove

(1) Press down on the skin and lift one edge of the dressing.
(2) Gradually lift the dressing edge from the skin all around the dressing margin.
(3) Slowly lift dressing from wound.

Frequency of dressing change

1–7 days depending on the amount of exudate.

Advantages

(1) The dressing is waterproof and washable.
(2) Good adhesion.

Disadvantages

(1) Slight odour at dressing change.
(2) Skin will become macerated if the exudate becomes heavy.

TIELLE ®

Description

A foamed gel dressing comprising four layers: an absorbant polyurethane central island; a non-woven wicking layer; an adhesive layer; and a waterproof, semi-permeable backing layer.

Sizes

11 cm × 11 cm.

Indications

Low to moderately exuding wounds.

Contraindications

Infected wounds.
Heavily exuding wounds.

How to apply

(1) Cleanse wound and dry skin around.

(2) Remove backing paper and apply Tielle to the wound, ensuring the wound is completely covered by the central island.

(3) If the wound is larger than the central island, a second dressing may be used to overlap the first.

Supplementary dressings

None.

How to remove

(1) Lift a corner of the dressing and gently peel back from the wound.

Frequency of dressing change

Up to 7 days depending on the amount of exudate.

Advantages

(1) Easy to apply.

Disadvantages

(1) Only one size available.

TRANSITE ™

Description

Two layers of plastic film bonded together. One layer is hydrophilic and the other hydrophobic. The film has a series of narrow slits arranged in rows.

Sizes

10 cm × 10 cm; 15 cm × 20 cm; 30 cm × 40 cm.

Indications

Donor sites.
Partial- and full-thickness burns.

Contraindications

Infected wounds.
Wounds with necrotic eschar.

How to apply

(1) Cleanse wound and dry skin around.
(2) Select a suitable size to allow a 2–3 cm margin around the wound.
(3) Remove the backing paper from one of the white handles and fix in position on one side of the wound.
(4) Remove the main backing paper without stretching the dressing and apply to wound.
(5) Remove the backing paper from the second handle and fix in place.

Supplementary dressings

Absorbent pad (to soak up exudate).
Tape or bandage.

How to remove

(1) Lift a corner of the dressing and gently peel from wound.

Frequency of dressing change

Change outer dressing as needed. Transite can be left in place until the wound is healed or it falls off.

Advantages

(1) Responds to the varying amounts of exudate.
(2) Can be left in place until wound heals.

Disadvantages

(1) Care needed to avoid stretching the dressing on application as this will alter the function of the slits.

VARIDASE ™

Description

A sterile powder containing streptokinase and streptodornase.

Sizes

1 vial + 20 ml of normal saline.

Indications

Necrotic tissue.
Infected slough.

Contraindications

Active haemorrhage.
Granulating and epithelializing wounds.

How to apply

(1) Cleanse wound and dry skin around.
(2) Reconstitute the powder, avoiding frothing and shaking.
(3) Varidase may be applied in several ways: soak gauze and cover with a semi-permeable film to prevent drying out; cross-hatch necrotic eschar to allow enzymes to penetrate; injected under necrotic eschar; mixed with 5 ml of saline and 15 ml of an inert gel and applying to the wound.

Supplementary dressings

Gauze.
Semipermeable film.

How to remove

(1) Loosen and remove outer dressings.
(2) Wash any remaining dressing from wound.

Frequency of dressing change

1–2 times daily.

Advantages

(1) Will rapidly remove necrotic eschar.

Disadvantages

(1) Expensive.
(2) Requires frequent dressing change.

VIGILON ™

Description

An inert hydrogel containing 96% water and 4% cross-linked polyethylene oxide.

Sizes

7.5 cm × 15 cm; 10 cm × 10 cm; 7.5 cm × 20 cm; 15 cm × 20 cm.

Indications

Superficial wounds with moderate to low exudate.

Contraindications

Wounds with necrotic eschar.
Infected wounds.
Wounds with heavy exudate.

How to apply

(1) Cleanse wound and dry skin around.
(2) Select a suitable size to cover wound.
(3) Remove the protective outer film from one side of the dressing and position exposed side of dressing onto the wound.
(4) The remaining film layer may be left in place as an occlusive dressing or removed.

Supplementary dressings

Absorbent pad.
Bandage or tape.

How to remove

(1) Loosen and remove outer dressings.
(2) Lift Vigilon from wound.

Frequency of dressing change

1–3 days depending on the amount of exudate.

Advantages

(1) Soothing, cool feeling to wound.

Disadvantages

(1) Expensive.
(2) Dehydrates quickly.

Appendix B
Pressure-Relieving Mattresses and Beds

AIR MATTRESSES AND BEDS

Type of mattress	Trade names	Description
Static air mattress	Airtech Topper Carelite II First Step Waffle Floatation System	These overlays are intended for use over a standard mattress. Inflated by hand or electric pump.
Dry floatation air mattress	Roho Pressure Cradle	This is a more sophisticated static air mattress. The patient lies *in* rather than on it.
Alternating air mattress	Alpha X-cell Astec B.A.S.E. Bubble Pad Biwave Plus Intercell Mattress Trancell Pad	Electrically operated, this consists of a series of cells arranged in rows. Each row alternatively inflates and deflates. The cells may be oval or wide.
Sequential alternating air mattress	B.A.S.E. PPS 2000 Quattro	These mattresses may have two layers of cells. They alternately inflate and deflate in a sequential mode, varying according to the model.

Type of patient	Advantages	Disadvantages	Comments
Low-medium risk	Cheap, easy to clean, folds flat to store.	Easy to get too much or too little air in the mattress.	Reduces pressure.
High risk	No maintenance costs, easy to clean	Relatively expensive, can be filled with too much air.	Reduces pressure and shear.
Medium risk	Quite cheap, easy to clean.	Air pipes may be easily disconnected on some models. Maintenance required.	Reduces pressure. Original version (known as 'ripple mattress) now discredited as the narrow cells increased pressure.
Medium risk, some high risk	Easy to clean.	Training needed to use effectively. Maintenance required.	Remove ordinary mattress, or bed becomes too high.

Type of mattress	Trade name	Description
Dynamic floatation mattress	Nimbus	A sophisticated mattress, consisting of 8-shaped cells. A sensor pad detects weight of patient and adjusts pressures accordingly. Cells alternately inflate and deflate in dynamic mode or can be turned to static mode.
Airwave system	Pegasus	A sophisticated mattress which has two layers of cells working in unison. They function in groups of three – one inflated, one partially inflated, one deflated.
Low air loss mattress	Alamo Clinirest OSA 1000 Paragon Convertible Biomed X	Works on the same principle as the bed. However, this system can be used with a conventional hospital bed and is portable.
Low air loss bed	BioDyne II Kinair III Low Flow Therapy Mediscus Paragon 3500 Therapulse Acucare	The patient is supported on a series of air sacs which constantly lose a controlled amount of air. The bed frame is articulated and electrically controlled, thus allowing easy movement of the patient.

Type of patient	Advantages	Disadvantages	Comments
High risk	It can be detached from pump to move patient from ward. Easy to clean.	Training needed to use effectively. Maintenance required.	Effective for patients with severe pressure sores.
High risk	It can be detached from power unit to move patient from ward. Easy to clean.	Training needed to use effectively. Maintenance required.	Effective for patients with severe pressure sores.
High risk	Portable. Cheaper than the bed version.	Still quite heavy to move Expensive. Training and maintenance required.	Probably not as effective as the bed version. But still gives good pressure relief.
High risk	Useful for difficult to move patients. Reduces need to turn patient.	Bed is rather high. Training and maintenance required. Expensive.	Some models have special function to improve pulmonary function.

Type of mattress	Trade name	Description
Air fluidized bed	Clinitron FluidAir Plus Polytron 100 Paragon 5000 Redactron	The patient 'floats' on a tank of ceramic beads through which air constantly circulates. This ensures very low interface pressures.

BEAD MATTRESSES

Type of mattress	Trade name	Description
Bead overlay	Bay Jacobson	The overlay is sewn into segments and filled with polystyrene granules. Vapour permeable water resistant cover.
Bead pillows	Paraglide	Consists of a series of transverse bead-filled pillows which conform to the patient's shape. Vapour permeable water resistant cover.

FOAM MATTRESSES

Type of mattress	Trade name	Description
Foam overlays	Modular Pro Pad Pressure Guard Lyopad	The foam is partially cut through in either cubes or channels to enhance pressure relief. Vapour-permeable water-resistant cover.

Type of patient	Advantages	Disadvantages	Comments
High risk	Useful for critically ill patients as they need not be moved.	Expensive to hire. Training required.	Mostly used in ITUs, major injury units or burns units.

Type of patient	Advantages	Disadvantages	Comments
Low risk	Easy to use. Does not raise height of the bed.	Not suitable for very heavy patients as the granules flatten.	Reduces pressure.
Low-medium risk	Versatile. Easy to move patients.	Training needed.	Reduces tissue distortion and shear.

Types of patient	Advantages	Disadvantages	Comments
Low-medium risk	Easy to use. Cheap.	Raises the height of fixed height beds.	Reduces pressure.

Type of mattress	Trade name	Description
Foam mattress	Cubifloat Omnifoam Plus Preventix Softfoam Transfoam Vaperm	A full-size replacement mattress made of different densities of foam.

GEL MATTRESSES

Type of mattress	Trade name	Description
Gel pads	Action Pads Tendercare	Pads of gel with an integral cover. They come in a range of sizes.
Gel mattress	Charnwood LDC	A full-size mattress with both gel and foam components.

HOLLOW CORE FIBRE PADS

Type of mattress	Trade name	Description
Hollow core fibre	Bodypillo Charnwood Comfort Permaflow Permalux Hygeiarelief Snuggledown Spenco Superdown Surgic goods Transoft	Hollow core fibre within a cotton cover. The fibre may be in the form of bolsters which can be individually removed. Vapour-permeable, water-resistant cover.

Type of patient	Advantages	Disadvantages	Comments
Medium risk	Easy to use.	Once the bed is made not easy to differentiate from standard mattress.	Reduces pressure.

Type of patient	Advantages	Disadvantages	Comments
Low-medium risk	No maintenance. No training.	Heavy to move.	Disperses pressure.
Medium risk	Easy to use.	Heavy to move. Once the bed is made not easy to differentiate from standard mattress.	Reduces pressure.

Type of patient	Advantages	Disadvantages	Comments
Low risk	Comfortable, easy to use.	Life-span often reduced by hospital laundry washing at too high temperature.	Reduces pressure.

WATER MATTRESSES AND BEDS

Type of mattress	Trade name	Description
Water mattress	Ardo Elwa Lyco	An overlay which has a foam surround and a number of water sacks or pads.
Water beds	Beaufort-Winchester Guardian 1250	These beds are, in effect, a tank filled with water. The patient floats on the surface cover.

TURNING BEDS

Trade names	Description
Egerton Turning Net Suspension Bed LIC Turnover Bed Mini Co-Ro Treatment Table Paragon 9000 Turning Bed Technabed Egerton Turning and Tilting Bed	Most are electrically controlled. Some models may be preset to automatically turn the patient.

Type of patient	Advantages	Disadvantages	Comments
Medium risk	Simple to use.	Heavy to move, unsuitable for rehabilitation patients, some find movement difficult.	Reduces pressure.
Medium-high risk	Provides true floatation.	Very heavy, difficult to move patients, some patients feel 'sea sick'.	Reduces pressure.

Type of patient	Advantages	Disadvantages	Comment
High risk	Very useful for severely disabled.	Expensive, some larger than a standard bed.	Useful for homecare of severely disabled.

Glossary

Angiogenesis   The growth of new blood vessels.

Autolysis   Breaking down of devitalized tissue.

Cellulitis   Inflammation of subcutaneous tissue with localized oedema.

Colonization   The presence of bacteria on the wound surface.

Contraction   The process where the surface area of the open wound is reduced. This occurs during the process of reconstruction in the healing wound.

Contractures   Fibrosis in the maturing scar tissue which results in shortening of the scar.

Debridement   Removal of necrotic or devitalized tissue from the wound either surgically, chemically or by autolysis.

Dehiscence   The splitting open of a closed wound.

Diapedesis   The method by which white cells move.

Eschar   The thick, hard necrotic scab covering a wound.

Exudate   Fluid which collects in a wound due to increased capillary permeability.

Granulation tissue   Fragile connective tissue containing new collagen, fibroblasts and capillary loops. Often described as 'beefy' red in colour.

Ischaemia   Localized deficiency of the blood supply.

Maceration   Softening of tissue, often around wound margins. It is associated with excessive moisture and is susceptible to breakdown.

Necrosis   Death of a portion of tissue.

Phagocytosis   The engulfing and destruction of bacteria, foreign bodies and necrotic tissue.

Tensile strength   The maximum pressure that can be applied to a wound without causing it to break apart.

Index